Electronic Health Records
FOR DUMMIES®

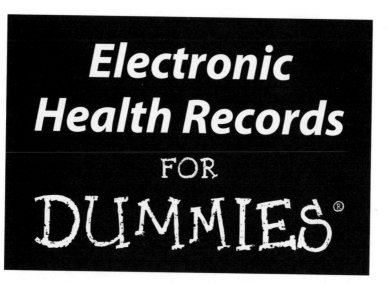

Electronic Health Records

FOR

DUMMIES®

by Trenor Williams M.D. and Anita Samarth

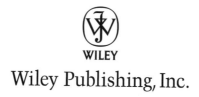

WILEY

Wiley Publishing, Inc.

Electronic Health Records For Dummies®

Published by
Wiley Publishing, Inc.
111 River Street
Hoboken, NJ 07030-5774
www.wiley.com

Copyright © 2011 by Wiley Publishing, Inc., Indianapolis, Indiana

Published by Wiley Publishing, Inc., Indianapolis, Indiana

Published simultaneously in Canada

For general information on our other products and services, please contact our Customer Care Department within the U.S. at 877-762-2974, outside the U.S. at 317-572-3993, or fax 317-572-4002.

For technical support, please visit www.wiley.com/techsupport.

Wiley also publishes its books in a variety of electronic formats. Some content that appears in print may not be available in electronic books.

Library of Congress Control Number: 2010941212

ISBN: 978-0-470-62365-7

Manufactured in the United States of America

10 9 8 7 6 5 4 3 2 1

WILEY

About the Authors

Dr. Trenor Williams is a family practice physician and co-founder and CEO of Clinovations, a healthcare advisory consulting firm based in Washington, DC. Over the last ten years, he has helped health systems, office practices, and physicians select and implement electronic health records in both the United States and abroad. He has worked with a number of EHR systems and is currently leading inpatient and ambulatory engagements at MedStar Health, Bon Secours Health System, and Adventist Health Care. He has significant experience supporting benefits realization, physician adoption, clinical transformation strategies, and working with third-party vendors to develop evidence-based clinical content.

Dr. Williams is Associate Editor of *Improving Medication Use and Outcomes with Clinical Decision Support: A Step-by-Step Guide*, which received the 2009 HIMSS Book of the Year Award. Prior to beginning his consulting career, Trenor was the Medical Director of Family Practice at Mammoth Hospital in California and was a Lieutenant Commander in the U.S. Naval Reserve. He holds a B.S. in Biology from Virginia Polytechnic Institute, M.D. from Marshall University, and completed his family practice residency at Kaiser Permanente in Los Angeles.

Anita Samarth is co-founder and President of Clinovations where she leads the company's public and non-profit sector work. She has more than 15 years of experience providing strategy, planning, management, and implementation consulting to over 60 clients in the area of health information technology. Her client organizations include large integrated health systems, hospitals, physician practices, federal government agencies, non-profits and NGOs, and state/local departments of health. She is currently working as the Technical Assistance Services Director for eHealthDC, the District of Columbia's Regional Extension Center for Health IT.

Prior to Clinovations, Ms. Samarth founded ASTECH Consulting, where she led projects for the Agency for Healthcare Research and Quality (AHRQ), Office of the National Coordinator for Health IT (ONC), and the Certification Commission for Health Information Technology (CCHIT). Ms. Samarth previously worked as Program Director for the eHealth Initiative, National Practice Manager for GE's EHR Clinical Consulting practice, Manager at First Consulting Group (now CSC), and Senior Consultant with Accenture. Ms. Samarth holds Bachelor of Science degrees from Johns Hopkins University in Biomedical Engineering and in Electrical Computer Engineering.

Dedications

Trenor Williams would like to dedicate this book to his family, especially his wife Sara and daughter Charlotte, for their patience, love and support as he worked way too many nights and weekends on this book.

Anita Samarth would like to dedicate this book to all of my mentors who have challenged me and expanded my skills through the years — you pushed and didn't flinch when I responded to assignments saying, "you know I'm an engineer, right?" You have helped me transform to who I am today.

Authors' Acknowledgments

The authors would like to thank the entire team at Wiley Publishing, specifically Kyle Looper, our Acquisitions Editor, for finding us and having faith in us to write this book, and helping guide us through the entire process. He took two *Dummies* novices and helped make this book possible with his patience and persistence. Thanks to Rebecca Senninger, our fabulous Project Editor, who worked tirelessly to help us continually improve the book. She put up with our work excuses and somehow kept us on track. Thanks to the team of copy and technical editors, including Brian Walls and Teresa Luckey, who brought their considerable experience and skills to help us along the way.

The authors would like to thank their Clinovations team including Billy, Greg, Jamie, Karen, Kevin, Lygeia, Rodrigo, and Ted who helped with research, editing, and extra work while both authors finished this book. Also, thanks to all of the Clinovations clients who gave us the opportunity to work with them. Your projects provided us the experience and knowledge necessary to write this book. You are the experts and we're extremely lucky to work with you.

A huge thanks to Jen Dorsey who worked with us to turn our thoughts, notes, and drafts into a real book. She exhibited unbelievable skill, patience, knowledge, wit, and determination throughout the endeavor and we would have been lucky to finish this book in another year without her assistance. You are a complete joy to work with and we truly appreciate all that you did for us.

Trenor would also like to thank his parents who have gone from saying "my son the doctor" to "my son the author."

Anita would like to thank her husband, Bob Filley, for his support during writing this book and putting up with her in general. She would also like to thank her family for their lifelong support and hopes that this book will help them finally understand what she does for a living.

Publisher's Acknowledgments

We're proud of this book; please send us your comments at http://dummies.custhelp.com. For other comments, please contact our Customer Care Department within the U.S. at 877-762-2974, outside the U.S. at 317-572-3993, or fax 317-572-4002.

Some of the people who helped bring this book to market include the following:

Acquisitions and Editorial

Project Editor: Rebecca Senninger

Acquisitions Editor: Kyle Looper

Copy Editor: Brian Walls

Technical Editor: Teresa Luckey

Editorial Manager: Leah Cameron

Editorial Assistant: Amanda Graham

Sr. Editorial Assistant: Cherie Case

Cartoons: Rich Tennant
(www.the5thwave.com)

Composition Services

Project Coordinator: Katherine Crocker

Layout and Graphics: Joyce Haughey. SDJumper

Proofreaders: ConText Editorial Services, Inc., John Greenough

Indexer: Palmer Publishing Services

Special Help

Jennifer Dorsey, Jennifer Riggs

Publishing and Editorial for Technology Dummies

Richard Swadley, Vice President and Executive Group Publisher

Andy Cummings, Vice President and Publisher

Mary Bednarek, Executive Acquisitions Director

Mary C. Corder, Editorial Director

Publishing for Consumer Dummies

Diane Graves Steele, Vice President and Publisher

Composition Services

Debbie Stailey, Director of Composition Services

Contents at a Glance

Table of Contents

Part IV: Optimizing and Improving Your EHR.............. 255

Chapter 14: Keeping Your Patients Healthy with an EHR.........257

Chapter 15: Directing Patient Access and Communication.......275

Chapter 16: Improving and Tweaking the System 289

Introduction

Welcome to *Electronic Health Records For Dummies!* Consider this your personal, private course in navigating the choppy waters of electronic health record (EHR) selection and implementation. The reach of EHRs is wide, affecting clinicians, physicians, hospitals, office staff, labs, billing and insurance companies, and even pharmacies. Although the topic can sometimes be overwhelming, you can handle it because you know your professional needs and your staff's. But, if you don't, you will by the time you read this book.

You'll find as you read this book that mastering the world of EHR is multi-faceted. You need to know what benefits you hope to receive from an EHR system implementation, how to analyze potential vendors, and how best to train you and your colleagues and staff. You must understand what you need; doing so ensures that you select the best vendor and product so you and your staff can spend more time working with patients and less time chasing down charts in a file room. Fear not; technology is friendly here. So stick out your hand, shake on it, and introduce yourself to your new best friend, the EHR.

About This Book

There is a world to know about electronic health records, and the volume of information can seem overwhelming at times. That is why we ground your EHR education in a healthy dose of background tempered with a massive shot of step-by-step how-to advice on the EHR adoption process. You get the story on what the EHR mandate is, what it means to the healthcare industry, and how it affects you, specifically. You view the landscape of what is available as well as receive information on help and oversight. You jump into content about planning for EHRs and how to implement them in the way that most benefits you and your practice. Finally, you look at how to optimize and improve your EHR experience. We even throw in some bonus top ten lists at the end that we hope you find useful.

Foolish Assumptions

We assume you are one of these people:

- A physician looking to move to a more paperless EHR system

- A medical professional in charge of managing a medical office, hospital, or clinic

- An aspiring medical information technology professional who wants to know more about how an EHR factors into the overall health IT picture

No matter what made you grab this book off the store shelf, we hope it will give you the background and guidance you need to make the EHR decision that is best for you and your colleagues. Choosing an EHR is like assembling a 1000-piece health IT puzzle. It takes a good dose of patience, a dash of IT knowledge, and a pinch of good humor. The EHR world is full of processes, procedures, and praxis.

How This Book Is Organized

This book starts at the most logical beginning — researching EHRs — and moves through the EHR process until your EHR and your practice are running efficiently.

Part 1: Health Information Technology Basics

In Part I, we provide you with an overview of what, exactly, an EHR is and does. You find out about the scope of the EHR: who uses it, where they use it, and why they use it. You also read about factors related to moving to an EHR, including how to consider your office infrastructure, figure costs and benefits, and research vendors. Chapter 1 discusses how this impending change will affect the people most important to your practice: employees and patients. Chapter 2 covers the different electronic recordkeeping options, including the typical EHR, e-prescribing, practice management and billing systems, and personal health records. Chapter 3 — all legislation, all the time — offers you basics about health information legislation and its impact on EHRs.

Part II: Planning for an EHR

In Part II, you consider your needs, research vendors, and choose your EHR. You find out about assessing your office's readiness for EHR selection and implementation, and crunch some numbers to determine the costs, benefits, and return on your EHR investment. After that, you read all about the complexities of surveying the vendor landscape and choosing the right EHR scenario for you. Finally, you read the fine print of negotiating and signing a contract that will dictate your new (hopefully positive) relationship with your EHR vendor.

Part III: I've Bought a System, Now What? Implementing an EHR

Now for the fun part — you get to play with your new toy. Part III covers what to do after you and your staff embrace the changes that electronic record-keeping brings. You will find that going paperless is a freeing experience, but it also presents new challenges, such as redesigning workflows, assigning roles and responsibilities, and training everyone involved. Therefore, we provide tips and tricks to transition your stakeholders (colleagues, clients, patients, and staff) into the new EHR system so that "going live" goes as smoothly as possible.

Part IV: Optimizing and Improving Your EHR

Part IV focuses on making the most of your EHR experience. After all, the whole point of the EHR is to make life in your office or clinic flow more smoothly. Here, you get some ideas about using the EHR to your patients' advantage and setting the EHR up to manage individuals and patient groups. You read about how you can set up patient-specific communication tools, such as alerts, messages, and personalized e-mail. Finally, you can use some of the suggestions in the final chapter of this section to tweak and improve the performance of your EHR over time.

Part V: The Part of Tens

Dave Letterman has nothing on these top ten lists. If brevity is the soul of wit (all apologies to Shakespeare), then consider the Part of Tens witty, indeed. Here, we cover Web sites to visit, pitfalls to avoid, and questions to ask while you're making the EHR move.

Icons Used in This Book

Don't be surprised to see small pictures dotting the pages of this book. Those little graphics are signposts for you to stop and take note of important information. Think of them as you would a road sign — something to read while you cruise along on your journey. Be sure to stop and look at these kernels of knowledge while you peruse the book:

The bull's-eye symbol signifies a great tip or trick that will help you choose and use an EHR.

This icon indicates things to watch out for, usually common mistakes people make when all there is to know about and do with an EHR overwhelms them. Consider these miniature cautionary tales.

This icon indicates something cool and perhaps a little offbeat from the discussion at hand.

This icon serves as a friendly reminder about an important bit of information that will help you in your EHR journey.

Part I
Health Information Technology Basics

The 5th Wave   By Rich Tennant

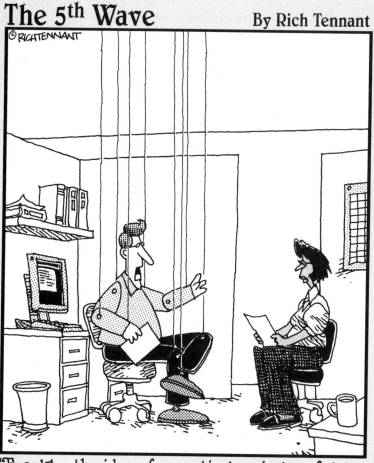

"Frankly, the idea of an entirely wireless future scares me to death."

In this part . . .

This book starts at the most logical beginning, the background of medical information technology. Chapter 1 gives you the background on the EHR — where it came from and why it's important to the healthcare picture. Chapter 2 lays out the fine print of what is available to you in the EHR world, and Chapter 3 walks you through how to find help and oversight by connecting with regional extension centers, government agencies, and hometown resources.

Chapter 1

Understanding EHRs

*I*f you're reading this book, you've already decided to at least consider taking the leap into the paperless world. That file room is looking mighty packed with paper, and you're starting to envision it as a nice, new break room or perhaps an additional exam room. You're keeping track of all the time it takes to pull charts, jot down or transcribe notes, and run back and forth from the fax machine. You think there has to be a better way to communicate with your patients and engage them in their care. You think it's time for a change, a change that streamlines your workflow, improves the quality of care you can deliver to patients, and clears up both physical and mental space for everyone in the office. It's time for the electronic health record; it's time for your EHR.

In this chapter, we give you a big picture look at EHR systems so you know what you're jumping into and walk you through the benefits you receive from one.

Recognizing the Worldwide Scope of EHR

To really "get" what EHR is all about, you first need to consider who uses an EHR and why, and what an EHR means to your practice. After all, you wouldn't buy a new car unless you did a bit of background research, right?

Well, maybe you would, but you might end up with a lemon. So, make this an all-lemonade, no-lemons experience and take a peek at what EHR is up to around the world. You'll be glad you did.

Checking EHR usage in the United States

Thanks to the continuing push for healthcare reform and legislation in the area of health information technology, physicians and clinics are going paperless at a faster rate, and the EHR market is going gangbusters to keep up with demand. Right now, there are more than 400 EHR vendors and counting, and they're all vying for a chunk of your business.

As you consider an EHR, here are some facts to think about:

- According to a 2008 article in *Pediatric News,* the goal of the federal government is to have 40 percent of all medical professionals using EHR by 2014.

- The Centers for Medicare & Medicaid Services (CMS) estimates that of the 404,000 eligible medical professionals in 2011, between 10 and 36 percent will adopt EHR in 2011, 15 to 44 percent will adopt in 2013, and 21 to 53 percent will adopt in 2015. In other words, EHR is big, and its usage is on the rise.

- A 2009 study by the Center for Disease Control and Prevention (CDC) states that 44 percent of medical professionals have already adopted a partial, basic, or fully functional EHR. Figure 1-1 shows the breakdown.

In 2015, Medicare will reduce payments for any physician not using EHR, so though it isn't technically required, your bottom line may thank you for adopting a system.

Looking at EHR usage around the world

The United States isn't the only country making wider use of EHR. In fact, several countries have already achieved widespread adoption of paperless systems. Four countries — the United Kingdom, Netherlands, Australia, and New Zealand — are tops in EHR usage with more than 90 percent of general practitioners using some kind of EHR system. Germany, too, is making progress toward electronic records, with between 40 and 80 percent compliance.

Some of these EHR gold star countries are also looking long-term to make more aspects of patient care management electronic. Australia, for example, is dedicated to creating a lifetime EHR for every citizen. HealthConnect is the major national EHR initiative in Australia, made up of territory, state, and federal governments. In New Zealand, more than 50 percent of physicians who use EHR also prescribe medications electronically in an attempt to make a full-scale move to electronic recordkeeping for all aspects of care.

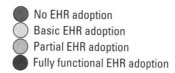

● No EHR adoption
○ Basic EHR adoption
○ Partial EHR adoption
● Fully functional EHR adoption

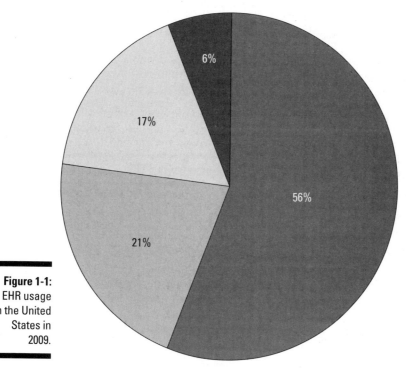

Figure 1-1:
EHR usage
in the United
States in
2009.

6%

17%

21%

56%

Knowing the Reasons to Implement EHR

So, great. Everyone else is doing it — adopting EHR, that is. "Why should I?" you ask. Well, the reasons for implementing EHR are as varied as the people who use them. Some physicians want quicker access to patient medical record information, whereas others want to interface more easily with other stakeholders, such as labs and pharmacies. However, the one thing every EHR stakeholder has in common is that they want to make their practices better by improving quality and streamlining their workflows. If we had to narrow the reasons to major categories, these would be (they are) at the top of the list.

Quality improvement opportunities

We don't know any physicians who don't want their patients to receive the best quality of care. One of the most vital components of that care is how information is shared with colleagues and staff, and how efficiently and clearly it's communicated with the patient. An EHR provides an opportunity to improve quality throughout the scope of the patient experience.

Because you can manage most aspects of your practice's everyday operations through an EHR, your workflow is streamlined, allowing for more quality time spent with patients. Where paper systems fail, EHRs excel, especially in improving information accuracy. Table 1-1 compares paper-based systems with EHR systems.

Table 1-1	Paper versus EHR
Inefficient Paper-Based System	*Efficient EHR System*
Paper charts are easy to misfile.*	Electronic files are fully searchable and backed up on a server.
Time is spent pulling charts and refiling.	Charts are updated and e-filed instantly.
Paper charts are viewed and accessed by one individual at a time.	Electronic charts can be simultaneously viewed and updated by multiple people.
Charts rarely include preventive care guidelines, which are often complex and difficult to commit to memory.**	Electronic charts can be linked to preventive care guidelines and updated as information changes.
Identification of patient characteristics is often difficult and time-consuming.	Patient characteristics are fully searchable and linked to patient history.
Clinicians must rely upon memory for clinical guidelines and decision support.	Clinical decision support rules can generate alerts for drug-drug, drug-dose, and drug-disease interactions.

Inefficient Paper-Based System	Efficient EHR System
Drug recalls are difficult to communicate and cross-reference with affected patients.	Patient files can be searched for medications, and flagged for drug recalls and updates.
Difficult to use for chronic disease management.	Clinical care guidelines can be available when viewing a patient's record triggered by clinical data.
Management of patient panels or groups is done manually or via patient registries.	Patient groups and panels can be set up and managed.
Handwritten or voicemail appointment reminders are sent each day by staff members.	Automatic appointment reminders can be sent.
Scheduling is coordinated by staff members.	Scheduling can be automated or performed by the patient using an integrated personal health record.
Insurance cards are copied, and information is keyed in.	Insurance cards are scanned and instantly put into the system.
Clinical encounter information is often transcribed and retyped into a chart, leading to human error.	Chart forms reduce the opportunity for human error.

*The Institute of Medicine (IOM) reports indicate that one in seven hospitalizations is because of missing clinical information.
**A 2003 study in The New England Journal of Medicine reported that patients receive only 55 percent of recommended preventive care services.

Getting rid of file rooms and missing records

Be honest — you're envisioning a sweet new break room in the place of that file room right now, aren't you? We thought so. That's what you can have after you move files to an electronic platform and lose the paper. New exam room, new supply closet, you name it . . . the space will be free to do with as you please. Employees will no longer have to spend precious minutes searching for and returning files or spend time performing file management, labeling, paperwork, and so on. The administrative time, from initial information intake to permanent filing, decreases by more than half when you use EHR.

Getting a new EHR means getting rid of stacks of folders and charts, which not only frees up more usable space for your office but also reduces the probability of misplacing records. Your staff will no longer have to spend time riffling around the office for Mr. Ferguson's file because everything they need to know about good old Mr. F. can be easily accessed through his EHR patient record. His file is never lost — it just lives securely online, saved on a backup server. Long story short, you're opening up space and saving a great deal of time by going paperless.

Getting information when you want it

Wouldn't it be great if you could access a patient's information remotely, say if you attend an out-of-town conference? Or, perhaps you need to quickly communicate medical history to a pharmacist to confirm accurate medication dosing. What if you wanted the latest lab results, but you can't seem to get through the intricacies of the lab's phone system in less than 30 minutes? Remember the last time you were on-call and received that annoying page at midnight? Wouldn't it be great to have access to your patient's information from your home so you could easily make the right clinical decision and then get back to bed? No matter the situation, your time is valuable, and you need patient information at your fingertips. EHR does that. You can pull patient info, set up instant messaging or e-mail alerts, and even (with some systems) get remote access to patient records from a PDA or smartphone device. Now that's something your musty old paper files can't do.

Looking at the Business Side of EHRs

Consider how, beyond improved patient care and better use of physical space, an EHR system will benefit you and your staff. The EHR is an all-encompassing entity that affects everything from scheduling and billing to workflow and patient communication. To think in a big picture sort of way, you need to consider three things: your office infrastructure and the viability of adding an EHR to the mix; the actual costs and benefits of adopting a paperless system; and the vendor landscape, such as who can provide you with the best EHR option.

Evaluating infrastructure and readiness

Think about how your current workflow, well . . . works. Consider the organizational structure of the office, and then ask who does each job and how each job is performed. Think of your office, if you will, as a city. The roads and varied transportation options act as critical components that allow you to get to and from work and social activities. Your practice workflows are the roadways of your clinic — if your office has potholes and road-blocking construction, you and your staff can't be efficient. You need strong background systems to provide a solid foundation for the people who live and work there.

Ask questions about everyone's workflow situation, from the top down, including

- ✔ Physician
- ✔ Physician assistant
- ✔ Nurse practitioner
- ✔ Nurse
- ✔ Medical assistant
- ✔ Lab technician
- ✔ Front office staff
- ✔ Filing or organizational staff
- ✔ Billing or back office staff
- ✔ Office manager
- ✔ Interns or temporary staff

 Have each staff member share a detailed description of a typical day, from the moment he walks in the door to the minute he closes for the night. Have each member include every type of patient or filing interaction he might typically have each day.

Then, ask yourself some big picture questions that encompass more of your corporate philosophy, including

- ✔ How is your organization situated in every respect — workflow, structure, culture, leadership, and so on — to welcome the move to EHR?
- ✔ How well do you know and understand your organizational and technological objectives?
- ✔ Is the move to EHR feasible and necessary for all aspects of your organization?
- ✔ Are all stakeholders, such as leadership and staff, properly positioned for success with an EHR system?

After you do some of that big picture assessing, you can begin to fine-tune questions about EHR readiness assessment in terms of corporate structure. These are good starting points for asking questions that can save you vital time and cash:

- ✔ How does your staff make decisions?

- ✔ How long does your staff take to make decisions?

- ✔ Where and how should decision-making be more collaborative?

- ✔ How does your staff communicate with one another? With colleagues outside the office? With patients?

- ✔ How does your staff deal with change?

- ✔ Do you have any organizational obstacles to a successful EHR implementation?

Compare the answers to these questions with the detailed workflow descriptions you get from your staff. In Chapter 4, we discuss more detailed readiness assessment activities and tools.

Figuring costs and benefits

After you assess the readiness of your staff to adopt EHR and figured out the cost of time spent working with paper charts, you can apply what you know to actual financial figures that help you put a real-life value on moving to a paperless EHR system. Here are some of the tasks that cost you real money based on time spent performing them:

- ✔ Speed of staff recording intake information

- ✔ Trips back and forth to file room or drawers

- ✔ Looking for missing files

- ✔ Duplication of work effort because of missing or incomplete files

- ✔ Time spent tracking down missing lab reports

- ✔ Prescription faxing and refills

- ✔ Chart pulls for phone calls, faxes, and follow-up

- ✔ Performing records requests

- ✔ Physician chart pulls

To figure the actual cost of day-to-day charting activities, add the number of minutes each staff member spends on those tasks and then multiply by the pay scale of that particular employee. No matter who performs the task, the cost is probably pretty high.

Although having an office staffer do some of this work might not seem expensive, saving him a few minutes here — or a moment there — adds up to real money that you shell out.

Other hard costs are associated with your "classic" paper-based system, and these are related to the money you spend on actual material goods and services. Consider the price you pay for

- The paper itself
- Folders
- Labels and stickers
- Square footage used for file storage
- Storage cabinets, tracks, and ladders
- Chart maintenance and replacement
- Copy or fax machine
- Toner and ink
- Hardware maintenance
- Billing paperwork
- Transcription services

Keeping all these hard costs in mind, think about what it might cost if you automated some or all these functions and jobs while eliminating the need for some of the material requirements that come with a paper-based record system. Numerous factors certainly affect your actual return on investment (ROI), and examining how you spend your money is a vital piece to implementing a successful EHR. In Chapter 5, we discuss how to determine the costs, benefits, and ROI of your EHR.

Numerous benefits to making the switch to EHR can't always be measured in dollars — these are *soft costs.*

Hard benefits are where EHR use directly correlates to that result in direct operating expense reduction or increase in revenue:

- ✔ Capture lost charges
- ✔ Increase preventive and management services
- ✔ Reduce claims denials and delays
- ✔ Reduce transcription

Soft benefits are where EHR use contributes to improvements that affect operating expenses or revenue:

- ✔ Increase physician productivity
- ✔ Increase staff efficiency
- ✔ Reduce chart pulls
- ✔ Reduce cost of chart storage and archiving

Checking out vendors and scenarios

After you assess your readiness and determine that you're ready for EHR, begin researching vendors. Create a game plan and timeline based on your needs and start shopping around for vendors.

There are more than 400 ambulatory electronic health record systems. The good news is that many of these vendor systems will work great for you and your practice, which takes a little pressure off feeling like you have to make the perfect choice. No perfect EHR exists; only the right one for your practice.

Products vary with their different bells and whistles, and many cater to a specific practice size or specialty. Thus, you need to develop your own requirements (see Chapter 6) so you can find an appropriate EHR fit for you and your team. Take time to talk with colleagues, your Regional Extension Center, specialty groups or societies, and hospitals in your area to get a feel for the vendor landscape in your geographical area or area of specialization. These groups have done their own research that you can benefit from and use as a starting point.

Don't feel pressured to fully explore each vendor. Instead, use your list of criteria to narrow the field and then focus your research efforts on, say, the top five that fit your needs.

One thing to consider comparing in terms of cost is the difference between server models. The first model is quickly becoming the most common approach for small practices — the *application service provider (ASP) model*, also commonly referred to as *software as a service (SaaS)*, is where an external party maintains and stores your practice's data. You can liken it to online banking where you have a relationship with your bank, and it provides you with online tools to manage your banking information. The other model is *site-hosted*, or the *client server model*, where your practice maintains the infrastructure for running the EHR application and storing practice data. For information on these models, see Chapter 4.

When you explore the vendor landscape, keep in mind that you need to ask pointed, specific questions about what the vendor provides in terms of functionality and workflow, information sharing, and training and support functions. Find out more about choosing a vendor in Chapter 6.

Prepping Your Practice for an EHR

Adopting and implementing an EHR requires a solid game plan. You can't just wake up one day and say, "Today's the day! I hope everyone will love the new EHR I bought for them!" You need to plan for the transition, map out a strategy for moving records to the new electronic system, and train your office staff. Think of the transition process as you might the weeks and months that lead up to the birth of a baby. You have to make room, clear out your old stuff, and mentally prepare for a new way of life. You'll hit some bumps along the way, but the result will be well worth the wait.

Embracing the required changes

Think of the approaching EHR changes in three factors: people, process, and technology. All three have to work together to successfully transition from paper to EHR. Ultimately, the whole transition process starts and ends with people. First, you have to get the stakeholders within your practice on board so they can get your patients on board with your EHR. Check out the nearby "Changing roles" sidebar to see how daily life might change for stakeholders within your practice.

Embrace the role of point person by making yourself available for questions and serving as both a liaison to the vendor and an advocate for further EHR training. Also, create a timeline of tasks associated with going paperless and help staff stick to the plan.

Changing roles

What has EHR done for you lately? Better yet, what will EHR do for you soon? Well, all that depends on who you are and what you do within your practice. Here's a small sampling of how your new life with EHR might change, depending on your role in the practice.

Physician, Physician Assistant, Nurse Practitioner

✔ Fully document all patient records, interactions, and recommendations.

✔ Submit prescriptions electronically and be notified of allergy, drug, and dose conflicts.

✔ Automate electronic prescription refills.

✔ Order diagnostic tests directly from the computer.

✔ Access clinical decision support or evidence-based guidelines.

✔ Access patients' records away from the office.

✔ Use tools for faster documentation.

✔ Use automatic health forms to quickly fill out required forms.

✔ Automate insurance eligibility checks.

✔ Query the EHR database to help manage patient groups.

✔ View and manage patient outcomes and quality of care delivery.

✔ Print patient education documents in multiple languages.

✔ Improve documentation for care coordination between clinicians and patients.

Practice administrator

✔ Assign tasks electronically and keep track of progress.

✔ Track patient wait times to create improved workflows.

✔ Automatically review staff productivity.

✔ Capture and store patient privacy notifications.

✔ Track access to patient files.

✔ Update and maintain access rules for each employee.

✔ Run reports on accounts receivable, earnings, reimbursements, and so on.

✔ Check and adjust claims immediately.

✔ Maintain records of patient insurance histories.

Nurse

✔ Manage patient calls and quick questions immediately from your location.

✔ Handle prescription questions online.

✔ Act on standing orders immediately, without getting verbal clearance.

✔ Run queries for continued care groups; for example, who needs flu shot next month.

✔ Use automatically filled e-forms to quickly fill out required patient forms.

✔ Print patient education materials quickly.

Medical assistant

✔ Enter vitals directly into patient records.

✔ Scan information provided by patients.

Front office staff

✔ Schedule all appointments electronically.

✔ Check for open time slots quickly.

✔ View schedules for multiple providers or locations on the same screen.

- Use instant messages to report patient calls.
- Fax directly from EHR.
- Scan insurance information.
- Use notes attached to patient records.
- Create automated checks for missing information.

Billing staff

- Generate automatic billing codes.
- Link diagnostic and CPT codes for more accurate billing.
- Submit, track, and manage claims.

- Keep track of patient co-pays.
- Create patient insurance history.

Patients

- View chart information and results online.
- Request prescription refills and renewals online.
- Communicate with clinicians using secure messaging or e-mail.
- Update demographic and billing information electronically.
- View and share clinical summaries between providers electronically.

Take a look at some of the possible functions that will likely change because of adopting an EHR:

- **Data migration**
  - Moving information from paper charts to e-records (via scanning and abstraction, mostly)
  - Maintaining paper records for reference, or as read only
  - Preloading data, possibly before formal EHR training
- **Training**
  - Participating in basic computer training
  - Participating in EHR training
  - Developing a training program for new hires
- **Financial**
  - Accounting for revenue lost during EHR training, implementation, and go-live phase
  - Creating a budget for software maintenance and support
- **Security**
  - Familiarizing staff with EHR security features
  - Setting up access to electronic patient information

- Setting up and maintaining passwords

- Educating staff about EHR security needs and requirements

- Installing and maintaining protective software

- Arranging for stronger insurance coverage of computer hardware

✔ **Back-up planning**

- Authoring backup plans if the EHR fails because of technical difficulties

- Setting up extra connectivity as a backup source of power

Providing for training and support

Training is a key component to your success with the new EHR. As you research potential vendors, keep in mind the training and support functions each prospect offers. Training is typically a two-fold process that involves some preliminary guidance with transferring and scanning files to the new EHR system, followed by a more formal training session prior to *go-live* (when the system is officially up and running). Check out Chapter 11 for more training info.

Your vendor relationship shouldn't end with training, though. You also want to use your vendor's support features and personnel throughout the EHR life, which can range from technical support to continuing education for you and your staff.

You have to stay on top of your office's training and support needs. Although vendors can provide a lot of assistance in these areas, it's your job to make sure they offer those things and stick to their promises. Follow up, always.

Communication is key: Before, during, and after

No one likes to be left in the dark, especially with office changes. So, be vigilant about sharing all the latest EHR developments with colleagues and staff as you move through the assessment, adoption, and implementation processes. From front office staff to physicians, keep everyone in the EHR loop as developments occur.

Show me the benefits!

Some of your EHR communication may involve getting colleagues and office staff on board with the migration to electronic records. The last thing you want is to drag people along grudgingly or to have them think you're adopting a system just to make sure your extra Medicare payments come through. Here are some EHR benefits to share with your fellow migrators:

- **Maximize, maximize, maximize.** EHR can maximize practice efficiency and reimbursements.

- **Burn that datebook!** EHR provides scheduling functions, including linking to other office systems (for patients with multiple providers), appointment reminders, and patient progress notes.

- **Stop memorizing codes.** Records of patient visits automatically generate a list of billing codes, allowing EHR to submit and manage claims electronically, limiting the need for follow-up.

- **Add up your extra minutes.** EHR reduces time spent searching for charts and missing files.

- **Everyone type at once!** Staff members with approved access can view or modify charts while others do the same. No more waiting for file access. Some systems can alert you when someone else is modifying a patient's record.

- **Feel free to take a real lunch break.** Why? Because you can access patient records remotely with EHR.

- **Instant messaging (IM) isn't just for kids anymore.** EHR allows you to send messages to staff and assign tasks to other stakeholders.

- **Link to other offices.** EHR allows you to order labs, receive test results, and even view diagnostic images in a flash. Many EHRs even link the results to patient records automatically.

- **Toss that nasty old clipboard.** You can help patients fill out information forms quickly with electronic templates.

- **Manage drug interactions.** EHR can flag patient records when drug recalls or interaction notices are issued, helping you keep patients safe.

- **Divide and conquer patient groups.** You can keep track of patient groups (diabetics, cancer survivors, and so on) to better manage their ongoing care.

Protecting and Serving Your Patients

Although all the benefits of EHR are terrific bonuses for you and your office staff, the largest stakeholder group to benefit from EHR adoption is your patients. By streamlining all those interoffice functions, such as charting and file management, the end consumer (the patient, in this case) benefits in multiple ways. Therefore, it's of the utmost importance that you always keep your patients in mind as you move forward through the adoption and integration processes.

Considering security and privacy

Security is a hot-button issue, especially in the world of medical recordkeeping. No one wants their personal, private healthcare information to get into the wrong hands.

As you review potential EHR vendors, prioritize security features so you can feel confident in telling your patients that their medical info is safe and protected. Some potential patient privacy concerns may include

✔ Who can view chart information (other physicians, lab techs, pharmacists, front office staff, and so on)

✔ How information is shared with other stakeholders

✔ What information, specifically, is found in a medical record

✔ How much other personal information is available electronically and to whom (Social Security number, insurance ID number, and names of relatives)

✔ What, if any, outside entities may request electronic health information (potential employers or relatives, for example)

✔ How information is stored and backed up

✔ How record access history is recorded to assure that only appropriate staff look at files

Sharing information as required and recommended

One of the most challenging aspects of your EHR adoption is sharing information that you're required to share and information that's in your patients' best interests to share. With EHR, several stakeholder groups — including patients, other providers, and state and federal organizations — expect you to share information. An atmosphere of open communication can get your patients on board with the EHR move and reduce their e-anxiety. Additionally, by providing key clinical information to other providers, physicians, and hospitals, you can significantly improve the care of your patients and reduce the opportunity for medical errors.

Include patients on the ground floor of EHR adoption by providing information about the upcoming changes and their affect on patients. Relay information in a variety of ways: signage in the office lobby and exam rooms, flyers, and communications sent with bills as well as engaging patients in conversation while you perform tasks. For example, you might tell new patients when they fill out their HIPAA form that, in the future, they may provide an electronic signature for HIPAA consent online.

Table 1-2 outlines some of the information that you can share and with whom you can share it based upon Stage 1 Meaningful Use criteria.

Table 1-2	Sharing the Wealth of Information	
Stakeholder	*Information*	*Stage 1 Meaningful Use Requirement*
Patients	Clinical summary that includes medication list, medication allergies, problem list, and diagnostic test results. Also, patient-specific education resources based on problem list, medication list, and laboratory test results	Provide electronic access in a "human readable" format via electronic media within 4 business days Electronically identify and provide patient-specific education resources to the patient
Providers	Clinical summary that includes problem list, medication list, medication allergy list, and diagnostic test results	Provide a summary care record for each transition of care or referral using the CCD or CCR standard
State and federal organizations	Quality measures to CMS, immunization information, and public health syndromic surveillance	2011: Submit clinical quality measures to CMS by attestation 2012: Electronically submit clinical quality measures to CMS Electronically record, modify, retrieve, and submit information to immunization registries Electronically record, modify, retrieve, and submit public health syndromic surveillance information

Your practice may be able to share more information than listed in the Table 1-2 with providers and patients, such as immunization history, treatment plans, procedure lists, or family history. We devote Part IV to sharing and accessing patient information with or from patients and other providers to better manage patient care. Work with your EHR vendor to set this up.

Such interactions don't have to be full-on tutorials; they can be simple asides or casual mentions about how the new process benefits patients.

Promoting wellness and disease management

Seeing how an EHR can improve patient care in the form of wellness and disease management is truly the fun part of the move. You and your patients can use some innovative features to make sure you manage their healthcare in a proactive way. What's even better is that your patients can finally become active participants in their wellness management in ways they (or you) never thought possible. Here are some useful ways the EHR promotes an active patient care involvement relationship:

- ✔ EHRs allow you to print and review patient education materials during the patient visit and provide access to electronic resources.

- ✔ You can create visual charts or graphs based on patient information that is entered into the EHR, allowing patients to see their health management in living color.

- ✔ Placing the computer where your patient can see it can allow a more open dialogue during the patient encounter. For example, you can say, "Mr. Ferguson, how about we take a look at your latest lab results together?"

- ✔ You can print a basic summary of the patient encounter for the patient to take home and share with family.

- ✔ You and the patient can view and confirm her history or medication list.

- ✔ You and the patient can view lab results or images together.

- ✔ EHR allows you to look up and discuss recent innovations in a patient's areas of concern.

- ✔ You can set up appointment reminders, prescription refill requests or notices, preventive service reminders, and lab test reminders in the format that best suits the patient's needs, such as e-mail, IM, a phone call, or a paper notice.

Getting your patients actively involved in their own care management is the cherry on top of the EHR sundae. When you can do that, you have everyone invested in your new world of greater efficiency, reliable quality control, and open communication.

Chapter 2

Understanding What's Available: The ABCs of EHRs

*T*ake stock of your office needs and determine what, exactly, it is that you want from the EHR experience. Right now, the EHR may be operating as a mere concept in your staff's minds, so to solidify it, you need to create a vision that includes your clinical and office requirements as well as patient needs. To do that, think about all those things in relation to what is actually available in the world of electronic health records.

In this chapter, we get you started evaluating your needs and your patient needs when considering an EHR.

Determining What Your Practice Needs

Everyone knows it's ill-advised to go into a grocery store without a shopping list. When you do that, you run the risk of filling your cart with all sorts of products that you don't need. Instead of eggs, milk, and bread, you end up buying a gallon of wasabi-flavored mayo (you saved by buying in bulk), a pummelo (because you've always wondered what it is), and a case of canned pumpkin (holiday baking *is* just around the corner, after all). So, although you feel completely prepared to make a boatload of wasabi potato salad and pumpkin pie for Thanksgiving, you realize that you have nothing to cook for breakfast today.

The same theory applies to the EHR. You really shouldn't go shopping for a new system unless you know what you need. Otherwise, you might end up with some glitzy features or a pretty interface, but little real-world functionality.

To determine your practice's needs, first think about what your practice is. Then answer these questions to get a clearer picture of what you want to get from the EHR experience:

✔ What is the case mix of your patients?

✔ What type of visit is most common for your practice?

✔ How many people work in the office each day?

✔ Does your practice have multiple physicians or just one doctor?

✔ Who constitutes the practice support staff?

✔ Who are the other clinical stakeholders with whom your practice interacts with frequently, such as consulting physicians, hospitals, and so on?

✔ Are employees part time or full time?

✔ How much time and how many resources are spent pulling and prepping charts for patient visits?

✔ Who is most likely to enter new patient information?

✔ Who is most likely to add intake information for existing patients?

✔ What information do physicians want to see or access quickly before they enter the patient exam room?

✔ Who is most likely to add post-interaction notations?

✔ Who monitors, manages, and notifies the physician of patient documentation (such as lab results, radiology results, hospital discharge summaries, consult reports, images, and so on) that arrives in the office by mail or fax?

✔ Who communicates lab results to the patient?

✔ Who follows up — appointment reminders, lab results, and so on — with the patient?

✔ Who handles prescription refill requests from patients and pharmacies?

✔ How does your practice communicate and resolve telephone inquiries?

✔ What do the physicians want most from an EHR?

✔ What do the support staff members want to do with an EHR?

✔ Where are the patient flow bottlenecks in the office, and why do they occur?

✔ Who does patient education, and when does this occur?

✔ What benefits does your staff want for patients?

✔ Are there any services you don't offer that could improve the patient experience?

✔ Would any functions that you don't have improve the quality of patient care or your practice efficiency?

✔ What billing issues do you want to improve?

✔ What issues do you have with paper-based coding and/or claims submittal?

✔ What's missing from how you interact with stakeholders outside your office, such as pharmacies, labs, hospitals, other practices, and so on?

✔ What does the current workflow look like for the physician(s), nurses, medical assistants, front office staff, billing staff, and so on?

✔ How do you manage diagnostic information, such as images?

✔ How comfortable is your staff with computers and technology?

✔ How many computers do you have?

✔ What kind of hardware do you have, and what could you eliminate (fax machines, for example)?

✔ Do you have space for computers and printers in exam rooms, work areas, and the front office?

✔ What processes seem redundant in your current paper-based setup?

✔ How do you categorize the services you offer (diagnostic, cognitive, and so on)?

✔ Do you want to offer more procedures in the future?

✔ What does your budget look like in terms of existing clinical or practice management software, hardware, and personnel?

✔ What costs do you want to reduce or eliminate?

✔ What is your budget for an EHR?

✔ How are diagnoses and charges documented and processed for each patient visit?

✔ When do you verify or reconcile appointments and associated charges?

✔ How do you process your Medicare and Medicaid claims?

✔ Are your claim reimbursements maximized?

This is not an exhaustive list of questions to address, but hopefully it gives you a starting point for your own laundry list of what your clinic is and what you do. When you can answer some or all these questions, you can begin to get a feel for what you want to change about your current paper-based records system.

When you review your answers to these questions, see whether you can chart some trends. For example, do coding errors keep coming up? If so, jot that down as something you hope to overcome with an EHR. Maintain a Things We Want to Change list and share it with potential vendors.

Knowing What to Expect from an EHR

If you want to handle virtually everything in the virtual world (pun entirely intended), you want the *full EHR experience;* you can do any necessary recordkeeping, charting, prescribing, and communicating with an EHR system. In brief, you can do the following with an EHR:

- ✔ Enter and access all patient information directly into one, easy-to-access file.
- ✔ Integrate all major components of clinical practice in the short term (why a patient has scheduled a visit) and long term (figuring out a treatment plan).
- ✔ Reduce errors based on handwriting or miscommunication.
- ✔ Allow approved stakeholders to access patient records, both in-office and remotely.
- ✔ Create more streamlined workflows.
- ✔ Prescribe drugs without making time-consuming phone calls or managing faxes.
- ✔ Utilize clinical decision support functionality to improve quality and patient safety such as alerts, reminders, documentation templates, clinical guidelines, order sets, patient education materials, patient reporting, and quality dashboards.
- ✔ Prescribe drugs without making time-consuming phone calls or managing faxes.
- ✔ Engage patients in managing their care.
- ✔ Create long-term treatment and health management plans for patients.

- Manage groups of patients.

- Flag patient files for drug recalls, drug interactions, or helpful follow-up suggestions.

- Organize communications and messages among everyone in the practice.

- Integrate with billing and claims data or systems.

The EHR is not the all-seeing, all-knowing big brother in the sky; it's designed by humans, for humans. Therefore, an EHR can't do absolutely everything for you (sorry, it can't order takeout). The EHR doesn't know your workflow, and neither do vendor trainers. Trainers know how to implement their software and then train you to use it. So you have to communicate with them about your specific workflow issues.

You can narrow your EHR wish list a bit to focus more clearly on some of those big picture needs, such as improving efficiency, streamlining work-flows, strengthening communication among practitioners, and creating stronger patient interaction and quality of care. Figure 2-1 shows how an EHR can work with your needs.

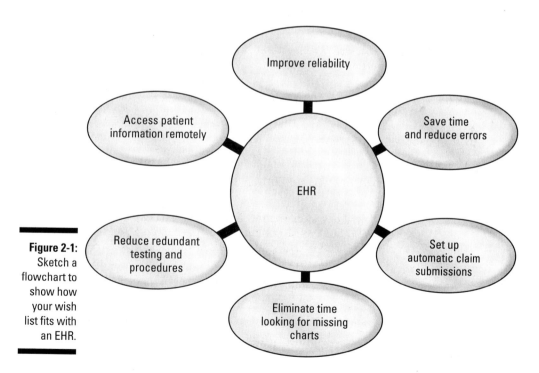

Figure 2-1: Sketch a flowchart to show how your wish list fits with an EHR.

For example, you can increase efficiency in terms of practice management by using the EHR to link all your scheduling systems, which allows physicians and office staff to link upcoming appointments to lab results or progress notations. You can also

- Save time and reduce errors by setting up the EHR to generate billing codes based on physician notes.
- Set up automatic claim submissions.
- Eliminate time spent looking for missing charts or information.
- Reduce redundant testing and procedures by using centralized information.
- Access patient information remotely with less time.
- Circumvent the problems associated with poor handwriting by typing or transcribing notes directly.
- Utilize standardized templates to improve the speed and accuracy of your documentation.
- Use superbilling features to describe services more effectively.
- Improve reliability of documentation with automatic coding features.
- Track pay for performance (P4P) measures like cervical cancer screening.
- Eliminate transcription costs.

Increased efficiency works hand in hand with streamlined workflows, allowing everyone in the office to do their jobs more smoothly. In the past, employees may have gotten caught up in the shuffling, filing, and searching for paperwork. But now, with an EHR, those elements are virtually nonexistent. Here are some ways your workflows can improve:

- Capture and file information instantly instead of dealing with note-taking and transcribing.
- Automate interactions with insurance companies.
- Order lab tests and receive results online.
- Link diagnostic images to patient records, which eliminates filing and searching for images and sharing data less effectively.
- Use templates to fill out forms automatically.
- Link to outside entities to receive information about drug recalls, health advisories, and disease information.

An EHR makes your workflows smoother and allows for stronger communication in the office and with colleagues in other locations, such as lab technicians, pharmacists, and specialists. EHR adoption improves your communication by helping you

- ✔ Allow multiple employees to view patient charts at the same time.

- ✔ Assign tasks to other employees or outside stakeholders electronically and immediately using notifications or instant messages.

- ✔ Share lab results or diagnostic images with fellow colleagues.

- ✔ Coordinate scheduling of in-office follow-up visits and referral visits to other clinics or hospitals.

- ✔ Access drug interaction information remotely.

Improved information sharing is truly a benefit of EHRs, but not everyone should be allowed to access patient files. You determine who has access to what (if any) portion of a patient's record. This not only protects the integrity of patient information, but it also gives you (and your patients) piece of mind that their health histories are in safe hands.

Perhaps the biggest big picture item on your needs list is improved patient care and interaction. After all, your patients are the end consumers of your day-to-day efforts, so you must meet their needs and your own. You can improve the patient care experience with an EHR by

- ✔ Setting up follow-up reminders about upcoming appointments, specialist appointments, upcoming procedures, lab tests, or prescription refills

- ✔ Using the EHR visual tools (such as flowcharts, anatomical diagrams and links to x-rays) to get a picture of a patient's progress or manage preventive procedures

- ✔ Capturing patient information more quickly, allowing more time for physician interaction

- ✔ Setting up patient group management to make sure groups of patients with similar conditions receive the same opportunities for treatment and continued care

- ✔ Connecting to disease management resources

- ✔ Printing resource information to share with patients

- ✔ Creating charts or graphs to help patients visualize their progress

- ✔ Printing a visit summary that's easy for patients to understand, take with them, and share with family or caregivers

- ✔ Engaging each patient with the EHR interface during their visit so they can feel more comfortable with the technology you use

The EHR versus EMR debate: What's in a name?

By now, you've figured out that we use EHR consistently throughout this book. You may wonder, well, what's an *electronic medical record (EMR)*, and what is the difference? Well, the answer to that question is a little different depending upon who you ask. People are in a few camps, but because you're reading this book, here's our answer: *Nothing!*

That's mostly true; however, EMR is used heavily in the ambulatory setting. In April 2008, the Office of the National Coordinator for Health Information Technology (an office within the United States Department of Health and Human Services that we talk more about later) commissioned a project that resulted in a *Defining Key Health Information Technology Terms* report.

The main difference between EHR and EMR cited in this report is that the EMR is used by and within a single organization (such as an ambulatory physician practice), and EHR applies when it contains data from or is accessed by multiple organizations. Here are the specific definitions:

✔ **EMR:** An electronic record of health-related information on an individual that can be created, gathered, managed, and consulted by authorized clinicians and staff within one health care organization.

✔ **EHR:** An electronic record of health-related information on an individual that conforms to nationally recognized interoperability standards and that can be created, managed, and consulted by authorized clinicians and staff across more than one health care organization.

The point is not to get too caught up in the proper use of these terms. You need to evaluate EHR functionality for your practice on your own. If EHR meets your needs, don't worry about whether it's called EHR or EMR. That's our story, and we're sticking to it.

Before the confusion over EHR or EMR has you singing about potatoes and tomatoes *à la* Ella Fitzgerald and Louis Armstrong and crooning, "Let's call the whole thing off," focus on two basic concepts:

✔ Know the capabilities of the system.

✔ Know what's considered your legal medical record and legal documentation for a patient and patient encounter.

That may seem like a lot of stakeholder needs to consider — and it is! But remember that in order for the EHR adoption and implementation processes to be meaningful for employees and patients, your attention to these multiple needs isn't just recommended; it's absolutely necessary. Complete EHRs can serve all these needs (and more), so if you have multiple concerns in various areas about how you operate, go for the full package deal and convert wholesale to an EHR.

Getting Your Feet Wet in Preparation for the Complete EHR

If you're thinking EHR is too much for you to handle, you may want to consider a few other options.

In 2011 or 2012, you can adopt an EHR for the full federal incentive payment of $44,000; in 2013, you can still qualify for $39,000. If you're eligible for the Medicaid incentive payment, you have even longer to qualify for the full $63,750.

Electronic prescribing

You can opt for electronic prescribing (or *e-prescribing*), either in addition to a standard EHR or as a solo act. If you plan to seek the federal incentive payment, e-prescribing is required, so it's a good first step in getting your staff used to an electronic workflow, and it can help support a number of improved workflows and support medication safety.

E-prescribing allows you to send, confirm, and refill prescriptions safely and quickly to participating pharmacies online. No more faxes, no more maze of phone calls, and no more checking back and forth to confirm drug interaction and dosage issues. Now, after a physician writes a script, it is sent electronically to the pharmacy of the patient's choice and get on with your life. We talk more about implementation considerations for e-prescribing throughout this book, particularly in Chapter 9.

A number of cost-effective stand-alone solutions exist for e-prescribing. In addition, each U.S. state and territory has received federal funding to promote access to health information technology; e-prescribing is specified on this list as a priority area for states to support. Health plans are getting in on this action, too. For example, Capital BlueCross deployed a stand-alone e-prescribing solution to more than 1,000 practitioners in Pennsylvania. Many e-prescribing solutions can also run on a handheld, mobile, or personal digital assistant (PDA) device, so you don't need to equip each exam room with a computer just yet.

You can do some other really functional tasks with e-prescribing, such as set up notifications to remind you and patients of upcoming refills, use alert features to notify you of drug recall information, and request drug interaction or allergy notifications.

The patient also benefits from e-prescribing because he can't lose his prescriptions, which he might have with a paper copy that must be hand-delivered to the pharmacy. The system can also be set up to accept only prescriptions that are covered by the patient's insurance, which eliminates issues at the pharmacy checkout.

Practice management and billing systems

Your clinical and operational workflows are tightly integrated and dependent upon each other, so it's no surprise that your information technology (IT) infrastructure needs to be tightly integrated as well. Tight integration of your EHR with practice management (PM) and billing systems is essential. For all the useful and functional things you can do with an EHR to replace paper files, you have just as many benefits that serve your greater PM and billing needs.

PM has a lot more to do with people management than just managing how you use and share files; it can involve improving communication among staffers, creating stronger methods of communication with outside entities or patients, and setting up your office for financial success through accurate billing and coding. Setting up PM and billing systems allows you to

- Computerize current processes.
- Improve interoffice communication.
- Increase efficiency by helping you electronically assign tasks to various staffers.
- Chart staff output and productivity.
- Set up more efficient scheduling functions (such as setting up multiple appointments, coordinating appointments with specialists, viewing appointments for various providers simultaneously, and so on).
- Improve patient wait times.
- Store and access notes on patients about everything from special needs and issues to recurring problems with scheduling or insurance.
- Automate processes related to confirming or updating insurance coverage.
- Save time by submitting and tracking claims online.
- Eliminate coding errors that occur because of illegible handwriting.
- Reduce patient intake time by setting up automated forms.
- Perform multiple tasks online (such as faxing, messaging, and phoning).
- Track how often staffers view or edit patient records and track their actions.

Your partner in PM: The long-reaching arm of the MGMA

Take heart in knowing that several professional organizations focus on the needs of those involved in practice management, one of which is the Medical Group Management Association (MGMA) and its associated organizations. They can offer all kinds of resources, from articles about the latest PM news and developments to discussion boards and networking opportunities. Here are some of the MGMA groups to know:

MGMA (www.mgma.com)

Description: The MGMA is an association for office administrators and the leaders of medical group practices. The organization provides important educational and career development opportunities for its members including American College of Medical Practice Executive (ACMPE) certification, conferences, seminars, and webinars.

Benefits: Access to member community forums, white papers and current research, a job board, networking opportunities, a member support center, benchmark data, and discounts on books and products.

ACMPE: www.mgma.com/about/default.aspx?id=242

Description: The American College of Medical Practice Executives (ACMPE) is the arm of MGMA that sets standards for the industry and promotes the professional development of PM leaders.

Benefits: Offers information on what it means to be a practice management professional, outlines governing rules and guidelines, and provides information about core values and principles for medical practice executives.

The MGMA Center for Research: www.mgma.com/about/default.aspx?id=778

Description: The MGMA Center for Research does what is fairly self-explanatory — it does research. This is the research and development arm of MGMA, and the group's Web site provides useful links to current projects and research initiatives. On the research docket right now are initiatives exploring patient safety tools, disaster and emergency preparedness, financial growth, and physician Medicare compensation. Think of this as the group that performs cutting-edge research that affects your day-to-day office life.

Benefits: Access to center findings, updates on current research and partner initiatives, and access to research resources.

Billing is a big part of the PM picture, and one of the areas that — we're guessing — you want to improve by setting up an EHR. Because the paper-based world can be rife with errors due to misfiling, coding, and good old humans, you probably want to reduce the margin of error that often results in lost profits. Some of your potential needs in the billing department might include

✔ Improving the amount and quality of documentation

✔ Quickly compiling reports on weekly or monthly charges and receivables

✔ Charting reimbursements in an easy-to-read format

✔ Setting up financial reports to reflect the information most important to you

✔ Tracking patient co-pays and deductibles related to in-office procedures

✔ Tracking claim statuses

✔ Documenting patient insurance coverage in a quick view format

✔ Reducing the number of days between claim submission and payment

✔ Setting up payment plans or special payment circumstances

✔ Linking family members' billing output to consolidate bills

Most practices already have some sort of scheduling, practice management, and billing processes and systems in place — some may be paper-based, via an IT system, or completely outsourced. If you don't have electronic systems in place, you need them. If you do have PM and/or billing systems in place, check with your vendor to understand what the vendor can and can't do in terms of integrating with different EHRs. We're sorry to report that a lot of legacy PM systems are in use across the country that really don't integrate well and aren't cost-effective to use with your EHR. A few implementation options are available:

✔ **Interface-based integration between a separate PM system and an EHR:** This is the most common solution implemented in the market because it enables integration of your existing or preferred PM system with an EHR, supports more of a best-of-breed approach, and can minimize disruption to front-office and back-office workflow. Talk to both of your vendors to understand prior experience in integrating these two systems because it makes a difference. Some systems have been interfaced many times, and the kinks have been worked out and all's well. On the flip side, it's never fun to be the guinea pig for the first time two vendors have interfaced a combination of PM/EHR systems.

✔ **Single solution with an integrated PM and EHR system in which your practice performs billing functions in-house:** Recently, we've seen this become a popular offering available from a single vendor that provides this integrated solution and also from EHR vendors that have partnered with a PM vendor to develop an integrated market offering of PM/EHR solutions. Having a single vendor or contact accountable for your integrated solution can definitely help reduce those he said, she said situations when it comes to system integration. Additionally, with an integrated solution from one vendor, it's much easier to pass the correct patient information back and forth between the clinical EHR and the PM system.

✔ **Single solution with an integrated PM and EHR system that includes billing capabilities:** Similar to the preceding option, this approach is gaining popularity and is being offered by both single vendors and by EHR vendors establishing partnerships with PM vendors. The difference here is that your practice's billing operations (including dealing with insurance companies) are also performed by the vendor. This is becoming an attractive model for practices that are cost-constrained or faced with the possibility of replacing their current PM system because the EHR payment model is typically a percentage of overall practice billing. In this case, the vendor is incented to maximize billing (as the laws allow) and keep accounts receivable to a minimum, so many practices see an increase in overall billing, which offsets the percentage-based cost of the integrated PM/EHR system.

Finding Tools for Your Patients

You might think that an EHR exists only to make your daily office life more functional. But remember that your most vital consumer — your patient — is a partner in the EHR process in many ways as well. Think of an EHR as a buffet of sorts. Everyone takes what looks appetizing to them and makes a meal from it. Similarly, multiple stakeholders can use the EHR to cater to their needs. Remember that an EHR can change the face of how you interact with patients, too, so their needs should be a piece of the puzzle when you research and select a vendor.

In April 2010, the California HealthCare Foundation released new consumer survey data, *Consumers and Health Information Technology: A National Survey*, which found that "Americans who have electronic access to personal health information know more about their health, ask more questions of their clinicians, and take better care of themselves." Take a look at some of the ways an EHR can address the needs of your most vital stakeholder — the patient.

Patient portals

No, a patient portal isn't a portal to another world or an alternate reality. A *patient portal* is a secure (thanks, HIPAA) online application that lets patients communicate with healthcare providers 24/7. Many EHRs offer a Web-based patient portal application that's linked to the provider's mainframe, so patients can be active participants in the management of their healthcare right along with physicians, nurses, practitioners, pharmacists, specialists, and even laboratories. Currently both the VA and Kaiser have the most experience with patient portals and more than 4 million Kaiser patients are connected to their health information and their physicians.

Regardless of what you choose to recommend to patients, remember that most portals follow similar guidelines and offer the platform necessary for patients to interact with other stakeholders. This isn't to say that patients can go into their records and alter, say, test results, but they can post new health developments (such as daily blood sugar numbers) or ask questions of their providers. Most portals allow patients to

- Complete forms online prior to an office or hospital visit.
- Request prescription refills.
- View their medical records.
- Review billing statements.
- Set up online payments.
- View lab results or diagnostic images.
- Schedule or change appointments.
- Communicate securely with providers.

Providing patients with access to their health information is a critical component to qualify for those federal incentive dollars, so you should seek a solution that's easy and seamless to your practice and EHR. We discuss patient portals in greater detail in Chapter 15.

Some portals are offered as part of the full EHR package, whereas some are set up as independent Web sites that link to EHR. For ease of accessibility, consider finding electronic health records that offer their own portal.

Most patient portals are linked only to one physician or hospital network. So if a patient uses multiple healthcare systems, he may have to link to more than one portal to fully manage his care.

After you choose and implement a patient portal, you can help patients get acclimated to their new virtual view of the healthcare world by offering assistance in the form of handouts, special workshops, or hands-on demonstration as time allows. You can also ease their tech fears by using online forms that mimic the look and feel of your traditional paper forms. To ease the transition on your end, consider adding the patient portal portion (say that three times fast) to the big picture a couple months after the go-live. After your employees feel confident about their EHR abilities, they'll pass that confidence on to patients.

You're the administrator of the patient portal, so it's up to you and your team to determine just how much information the patient can access. For example, interoffice notes like, "Mr. Jones is always late for morning appointments, so plan accordingly" can be hidden.

Personal health records

A *personal health record (PHR)* is exactly what its name implies — a record that keeps track of a patient's personal health history. Not to be confused with EHR (which is the documentation of the healthcare provider), PHR content is owned and, ideally, managed by the patient. There is a fair amount of confusion in the marketplace between patient portal and PHR, and the two terms are often used interchangeably, but unlike the EHR versus EMR debate, these two are materially different:

- ✔ **PHR data is managed and maintained by the patient.** The information contained in PHR can come from the individual and her healthcare providers and is made accessible to anyone the patient chooses. Like EHR, PHR is stored and maintained in a secure electronic environment. Though a patient can choose to make PHR accessible through the provider's EHR, it remains a separate entity.

- ✔ **Patient portals provide view only access to patient information contained in EHR.** The information in a patient portal is owned by the practice and can't be changed by the patient. Patient portals usually provide added functionality beyond view only access to health information.

As with anything else, when you talk with vendors about their patient access solutions, understand the capabilities and prioritize what makes sense for your practice; don't worry too much about whether it's named PHR.

Many of your patients may retain their health information in paper-based, PC-based, or Web-based environments, though many folks in the know are moving in the electronic direction. As shown in Figure 2-2, PHR and related solutions are available in all sorts of forms:

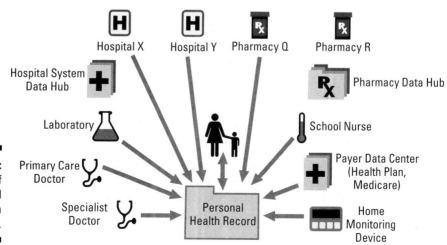

Figure 2-2: Sources of personal health records.

- ✔ Free, Internet-based applications that serve as conduits to manage health information, such as Google Health and Microsoft HealthVault.

- ✔ Web-based PHR that are tethered to an ambulatory practice EHR, offering more robust functionality than a patient portal.

- ✔ Many hospitals offer Web-based or PC software–based PHRs that provide linkages to certain hospital data.

- ✔ Health plans offer patient portals or Web-based PHR that include patient health and demographic information from health care insurance claims.

The result of some of that policy work stuff resulted in patient/family engagement as one of the five health outcome priorities for Meaningful Use of an EHR. (Translation: federal incentive dollars related to an EHR; we talk more about Meaningful Use in Chapter 3.) In January 2010, the Centers for Medicare & Medicaid Services (CMS) — the agency that provides federal funding for EHR adoption — included several relevant objectives in the proposed rule that was based upon comments from more than 2,000 organizations and individuals:

- ✔ Consumer's timely copy of, and access to, electronic records

- ✔ After-care summary for each outpatient encounter

- ✔ Discharge summary for each hospital stay

- ✔ Provide access to patient-specific education resources

- ✔ Complete drug formulary checking at the time of ordering

- ✔ Patient reminders for preventive and follow-up care

Remote patient monitoring

Remote patient monitoring is a cool tool for your EHR kit for primary care practices and practices responsible for managing patients with multiple chronic or complex conditions. You can address the needs of patients who can't always make regular physical visits to your office or who have chronic conditions in need of constant monitoring. Remote patient monitoring allows healthcare professionals to review patient vital signs, measure physiological responses, and communicate when physical distance prohibits office visits. Remote patient monitoring provides a cost benefit and improved quality to both practitioners and patients thanks to the ease of reporting and quick delivery of information. Doctors can monitor vitals and symptoms without the patient making an office visit, which frees time and office resources to manage patients who require more immediate attention.

Patients can use devices to track everything remotely from daily vital signs to disease- or condition-specific symptoms. Many devices are small and easy to care for; some can even be swallowed! Also, more and more electronics manufacturers are developing remote patient monitoring programs that work in conjunction with existing technology that people already use every day: smartphones, PDAs, PCs, and even cable boxes. So, you know "there's an app for that" somewhere!

Remote monitoring could include, but is not limited to, communication of

- ✔ **Physiologic measurements:** For example, weight, blood pressure, heart rate and rhythm, pulse oximetry, glucose, and so on

- ✔ **Diagnostic measurements:** For example, transthoracic impedance and so on

- ✔ **Medication tracking device information:** For example, medication pumps, infusion devices, electronic pillboxes, and so on

- ✔ **Activities of daily living measurements:** For example, ADL biosensors, pedometers, sleep actigraphy, and so on

Connecting to the Community: Health Information Exchange

You've determined your needs. You know what you want the EHR to do for your patients. All that's left is . . . everyone else. That's right, you're going global. Healthcare is, at its heart, a community effort. Everyone benefits from the expertise and experiences of everyone else. That's how people make strides in the fight against diseases like cancer, or develop new and innovative medical devices. People share, therefore they are. An EHR can help you not only share on a personal level (with patients) and a local level (with colleagues and staff); it can also help you share information across organizational borders to contribute to the global exchange of healthcare information.

A *health information exchange (HIE)* is exactly what it sounds like — healthcare information that's shared across organizations from varying hospital, community, or regional systems, as shown in Figure 2-3. By participating in an HIE, you can

✔ **Share patient data with other hospital systems.** Say, for example, one of your patients has an accident on vacation in a different part of the state. You can use HIE to communicate with the ER doctor who treats him.

✔ **Participate in continuity of care.** When a patient sees multiple providers, there is a likelihood that some providers won't be in your particular healthcare system. HIE allows you to communicate across system lines while maintaining the integrity of patient information.

✔ **Contribute information to public health entities.** Why is this important? Because epidemics are bad. The more information you can supply to groups, such as your local health department, the easier it is for them to chart the health of the population at large and prevent communicable diseases.

Several organizations offer support for providers participating in HIEs. Regional health information organizations (RHIOs) and state-level organizations provide information on terms and information exchange requirements as well as develop methods and standards for the exchange of health information.

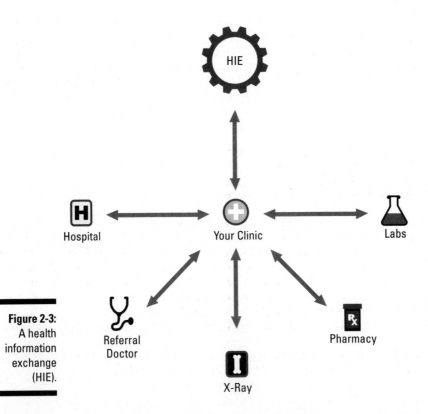

Figure 2-3:
A health
information
exchange
(HIE).

HIE

Hospital   Your Clinic   Labs

Referral
Doctor

X-Ray

Pharmacy

Chapter 3

Finding Help and Oversight

. . . .

In This Chapter

▶ Making sense of healthcare legislation

▶ Defining Meaningful Use

▶ Getting to know state and local healthcare organizations

▶ Standardizing EHRs

. . . .

*T*hankfully, you don't have to venture into the world of healthcare technology alone. A plethora of information — from federal legislation and state and local regulations to blogosphere opinions on the best EHRs for physicians — is available to help you choose an EHR. The trick, of course, is finding the most accurate and useful information. In this chapter, you get a quick course in how to find the help you need.

Checking Out Related Legislation (ARRA and the HITECH Act)

The American Recovery and Reinvestment Act (ARRA) has a wide-reaching affect on healthcare. According to the ARRA Web site (www.recovery.gov), the act increases federal funds for various programs by $224 billion and frees $275 billion for federal contracts, grants, and loans, some of which enter the healthcare sector. Additionally, a new level of corporate and government transparency requires that recovery fund recipients report how they use the money each quarter. Although governing legislation, you can think of the ARRA as a legislative body that's divided into subgroups and committees.

All data about how recovery funds recipients spend their money are posted on www.recovery.org. How's that for transparency?

Throw me a rope: EHR on a budget

Although the fed is urging that practices adopt an EHR, some physicians cannot afford adoption and implementation. Market dynamics can help you score a qualifying EHR (according to standards set forth by HHS) for a nominal fee or no fee until you receive your incentive payments. EHR costs vary greatly, but help is available thanks to the ARRA legislation. Here are some options to keep costs down:

✔ **Select an EHR offered or verified by your state or region's Regional Extension Center (REC).** The RECs are responsible for negotiating discount pricing with select vendors.

✔ **Select an EHR offered by your affiliated hospital or health system.** Many hospitals and health systems are extending their solutions and offering turnkey solutions for ambulatory EHRs for affiliated physicians.

✔ **Select an EHR vendor that offers Meaningful Use guarantees.** The burden is on the vendor to help you get your federal incentive payment.

✔ **Select an EHR vendor that offers you very low, if any, upfront fees via payment schedules.** You can delay payments until you receive your Meaningful Use incentive payment.

One of the biggest goals of the ARRA is to have all physicians and hospitals using computerized health records by 2015. Of course, the federal government doesn't expect you to adopt EHR just because they think it's a good idea; therefore, rewards and penalties address how physicians respond to the EHR mandate. Here are some ways the fed is gently coaxing providers that bill Medicare and Medicaid onto its EHR wagon:

✔ ARRA provides $19 billion to assist hospitals and physicians purchase and implement EHRs.

✔ The Department of Health and Human Services (HHS) promotes uniform electronic standards that will allow different EHR systems to work with each other.

✔ Medicare physicians who implement and use EHRs are eligible for a financial incentive up to $18,000 as of 2011 and a total of $44,000 by 2015.

✔ Medicare payments will be reduced for physicians who do not implement and use an EHR starting in 2015.

✔ Medicaid providers who meet the qualifying patient volume threshold will be eligible for a financial incentive up to $21,250 in Year 1 (starting in 2011) and a total of $63,750 by 2016, or Year 6.

To make all this EHR magic happen, the ARRA does what any good leader would — delegates. The people who govern ARRA also govern the Office of the National Coordinator for Health Information Technology (ONC) under the umbrella of the Department of Health and Human Services (HHS). ONC is charged with promoting the development of a nationwide health information technology infrastructure.

ARRA also establishes the Health Information Technology (HIT) Policy and Standards Committees made of public and private stakeholders who offer suggestions and recommendations on HIT policies and standards, implementation specifications, and requirements for EHR certification.

Portions of the HITECH (Health Information Technology for Economic and Clinical Health) Act are largely concerned with privacy and security issues that may arise while health records transition from a paper-based system to an electronic one. The HITECH Act allows for increased privacy and protection through HIPAA, ups the liability for noncompliance, and offers increased enforcement.

The HIPAA form that patients must sign to acknowledge they are aware of your participation in protecting their privacy may seem a bit outdated and rote. The reason for that is adherence to HIPAA (unless you get caught, which makes it fairly obvious) is difficult to enforce.

Thanks to the HITECH Act, patients must be notified of any unsecured breach of their personal information. Additionally, if the breach affects 500 people or more, the HHS must be notified. Such a notification automatically gets the breaching entity's name posted to the HHS Web site. In some cases (depending on the nature and size of the breach), media are also notified, presumably to make sure the word gets out to affected parties.

A security breach information notification is automatically triggered whether the breach occurred in your office or externally.

The HITECH Act obviously takes the privacy and security of patient information seriously. Similarly, patients' ability to freely access their information is of the utmost importance. Patients of physicians who have an EHR system have a legal right to obtain their electronic protected health information (EPHI) or designate a third party to do so on their behalf.

A small fee equivalent to the cost of labor may be charged to any patient who makes an EPHI request. So find out what that fee is, and let your patients know about it when you provide educational materials about your new EHR.

Do make your HITECH Act education a priority while you move through the EHR adoption and implementation processes because your bottom line depends on it. If you want to maximize your incentive funding and avoid penalties for noncompliance of security and privacy mandates, keep your ear to the ground for important new developments regarding the HITECH Act, including updates to HIPAA's privacy and security rules and regulations.

Introducing Meaningful Use

You will hear a lot of talk in the health information technology world about *Meaningful Use,* so become familiar with the concept. Meaningful Use means just what it says — Meaningful Use of an EHR technology. In other words, you are using the EHR for the purpose it is intended for: clinical documentation, improved quality, and improved patient safety in a manner that is in accordance with local, state, and federal rules and regulations. Though such a definition seems fairly self-explanatory, people still have a lot of questions about the specifics of Meaningful Use and several organizations continue to discuss and debate the meaning. Centers for Medicare & Medicaid Services (CMS) defines Meaningful Use as the use of health information technology to further information exchange among healthcare professionals and to further ARRA goals with three main components:

- ✔ Use of certified EHR in a meaningful manner

- ✔ Use of certified EHR technology for electronic exchange of health information to improve quality of care

- ✔ Use of certified ERH technology to submit Clinical Quality Measures (CQM) and other such measures selected by the Secretary of HHS

The EHR incentive rule proposes Meaningful Use criteria based on a series of specific objectives, with each objective tied to a proposed measure that all eligible professionals must meet to demonstrate that they are meaningful users of certified EHR technology.

The objectives are divided into a set of 15 "core" and 10 "menu" objectives. To receive the financial incentives from CMS, you must meet all 15 core objectives and 5 of the 10 menu requirements. You report the results for all objectives/measures, including clinical quality measures to CMS or to your respective state, through attestation.

The EHR incentive rule, brought to you courtesy of your friends at CMS, defines who, exactly, is an eligible professional who can be considered a meaningful user of an EHR. CMS defines a Medicare eligible professional as a

- ✔ Doctor of medicine or osteopathy

- ✔ Doctor of dental surgery or dental medicine

- ✔ Doctor of podiatric medicine

- ✔ Doctor of optometry

- ✔ Chiropractor

The term *eligible professional* widens the field a bit regarding who is eligible to receive Medicaid payments, and includes (in addition to the previous professionals)

✔ Certified nurse midwives

✔ Nurse practitioners

✔ Physician assistants at a Federally Qualified Health Center (FQHC) or Rural Health Clinic (RHC) led by a physician assistant

One group not eligible for incentive payments under the definition of Meaningful Use is hospital-based professionals (such as ER doctors or anesthesiologists) who provide the majority of their services in the hospital proper.

Don't know whether you qualify as a hospital-based professional? If you provide 90 percent or more of your services in a hospital, consider yourself in that category.

The government (via the EHR incentive rule) proposes a three-stage definition of Meaningful Use that will affect your incentive payments:

✔ **Stage 1:** You must capture health information electronically in a coded format and use the information to monitor clinical conditions, communicate the information for care coordination, and initiate reporting of quality measures and public health information. (See Chapter 2.)

✔ **Stage 2:** The government expands Meaningful Use in this stage by including parameters for disease management, management of medications, providing assistance to patients in accessing their personal health information, care transitions, communication with public health agencies, clinical decision support, and implementation of quality measures and research.

✔ **Stage 3:** This stage tentatively focuses on long-term strategies for healthcare professionals in the areas in Stage 2. Meaningful use will be demonstrated by planning for quality and safety improvements, working toward improved efficiency measures, adding elements of decision support for national high priority conditions, improving patient engagement by offering them tools for self-management of healthcare, providing access to patient data, and working toward improving health outcomes for the population at large.

Despite ongoing development of these stages, the discussion to define Meaningful Use continues among government entities, EHR vendors, and healthcare professionals; therefore, expect revisions to continue to make the final definitions of Meaningful Use flexible enough to accommodate a wide scope of healthcare professionals.

Useful Meaningful Use Web sites

Defining Meaningful Use criteria is an evolutionary process. You may wonder why because leading organizations and early adopters of EHRs have been demonstrating improvements to quality of care and patient safety over the last few years. However, there hasn't been much in the way of standardized reporting and guidelines. Despite strong efforts by the government, standards organizations, and professional organizations, added coordination was needed to make widespread EHR adoption a reality. Following ARRA and the HITECH Act, many government and private sector committees, work groups, and advisors are trying to piece together the EHR incentive program. Determining priorities, feasibility, and a reasonable "stretch goal" for the future takes time.

We've done our best to communicate to you the most current information, but we know that new data will be available by the time you read this book. Here's a list of helpful Web sites to find the most current information around:

Centers for Medicare & Medicaid Services (CMS) EHR Incentive Programs: `www.cms.gov/EHRIncentivePrograms/`

The Office of the National Coordinator for Health Information Technology (ONC): `http://healthit.hhs.gov`

Regional Extension Center (REC) programs: `www.HealthIT.hhs.gov/programs/REC/`

ONC Authorized Testing and Certification Bodies (ONC-ATCB): `http://healthit.hhs.gov/certification`

Agency for Healthcare Research and Quality (AHRQ) National Resource Center for Health Information Technology: `http://healthit.ahrq.gov`

Heath Resources and Services Administration (supports uninsured, underserved, and special needs populations): `www.hrsa.gov/healthit`

Because the concept of Stage 2 and Stage 3 Meaningful Use continues to change, start monitoring Stage 2 at the end of 2010 when the requirements begin to solidify. Communicate with your vendor, REC, affiliated health systems, professional organizations, and CMS to keep abreast of evolution and progression of these criteria.

Finding State and Local Resources

To make sense of all of this EHR-related information, you have several resources at your disposal. The goal of most of these organizations is to help you better understand the EHR mandate and its requirements, adoption and implementation criteria, and incentive structure.

Regional extension centers (RECs)

The federal government assists physicians in EHR by funding regional extension centers (RECs) to support physicians and their practices who implement EHRs in the next several years (see Chapter 6). Each REC, responsible for a geographic area, is expected to support providers in achieving Meaningful Use. RECs offer a menu of on-site, practical services to help you meet your EHR initiative goals. Initially, RECs focus on the primary care providers least likely to achieve Meaningful Use on their own, especially small practices with fewer than 10 providers and community health centers.

RECs focus on two target populations: physicians with an EHR who are looking to optimize their systems to meet the Meaningful Use criteria and primary care physicians who have yet to select and implement EHR. By working with your REC, you can get lower pricing through bulk purchasing agreements; access to implementation experts who provide advice on system design, workflow changes, training and support; and comprehensive sharing of best practices for a specific vendor and for general use of the EHR. REC fees range from free to a few thousand dollars, depending on whether you qualify as a priority provider, the range of services the REC is offering, and how the services are packaged.

The REC that covers your region is one of your best sources for information. Table 3-1 lists all the RECs. If you're not a priority provider for REC services, RECs have Web sites, printed materials, and other helpful resources to help you along the way. After all, they're helping many physicians implement EHRs, so take advantage of their experience and resources.

REC service offerings can be divided into three categories:

- ✔ **Adoption:** Vendor selection assistance, preferred EHR pricing, cost-benefit analyses, Meaningful Use education

- ✔ **Implementation:** Workflow optimization, go-live support, project management, IT support

- ✔ **Other:** Community forums, loan programs, lab interfaces, immunization registry integration

To contact the regional extension center in your area, visit `www.HealthIT.hhs.gov/programs/REC/` for the latest contact information.

Table 3-1	Regional Extension Centers	
REC Name	*State*	*Web Site*
Alaska eHealth Network	AK	www.ak-ehealth.com
Alabama Regional Extension Center	AL	www.al-rec.org
HIT Arkansas	AR	www.hitarkansas.com
Arizona Health-e Connection (AzHeC)	AZ	www.azhec.org
CalHIPSO (North)	CA	www.calhipso.org
CalHIPSO (South)	CA	www.calhipso.org
CalOptima Foundation	CA	www.caloptima.org
HITEC-LA	CA	http://hitec-la.org
Colorado Regional Extension Center (CORHIO)	CO	www.corhio.org
eHealth Connecticut	CT	www.ehealthconnecticut.org
eHealth DC	DC	www.ehealthdc.org
National Indian Health Board (NIHB)	DC	www.nihb.org
Quality Insights of Delaware	DE	www.qide.org/de
Rural and North Florida Regional Extension Center	FL	www.chcalliance.org/Services/RegionalExtensionCenter.aspx
South Florida Regional Extension Center Collaborative	FL	www.southfloridarec.org
University of Central Florida	FL	www.med.ucf.edu/rec/
University of South Florida	FL	http://health.usf.edu/paperfree/index.htm
Morehouse School of Medicine	GA	www.msm.edu/research/research_centersandinstitutes/research_cni_NCPC.aspx
Hawaii Health Information Exchange	HI	www.hhie.org
IFMC Health Information Technology Regional Extension Center (Iowa HITREC)	IA	www.IowaHITREC.org

REC Name	State	Web Site
Illinois Health Information Technology REC (Il-HITREC)	IL	www.ilhitrec.org
Chicago Health Information Technology REC (CHITREC)	IL	www.chitrec.org
Purdue University	IN	www.ihitec.purdue.edu
Kansas Foundation for Medical Care, Inc. (KFCM)	KS	www.kfmc.org/rec
University of Kentucky Research Foundation	KY	www2.ca.uky.edu
REC for Health IT in Mississippi	MS	www.eqhealthsolutions.com
Louisiana Health Care Quality Forum	LA	www.lhcqf.org
MA Technology Corporation	MA	http://masstech.org
Chesapeake Regional Information System for Our Patients	MD	www.crisphealth.org
HealthInfoNet	ME	www.hinfonet.org
Michigan Center for Effective IT Adoption (M-CEITA)	MI	www.mceita.org
Regional Extension Assistance Center for HIT (REACH)	MN	www.khareach.org
Missouri HIT Assistance Center	MO	www.assistancecenter.missouri.edu
Mountain Pacific Quality Health Foundation (MPQHF)	MT	www.mpqhf.org
University of North Carolina at Chapel Hill	NC	www.med.unc.edu/ahec
Wide River Technology Extension Center	NE	www.widerivertec.org
Massachusetts eHealth Collaborative	NH	www.maehc.org
New Jersey Institute of Technology	NJ	www.njit.edu
LCF Research	NM	www.lcfresearch.org
NYC REACH	NY	www.nycreach.org

(continued)

Table 3-1 *(continued)*

REC Name	State	Web Site
New York eHealth Collaborative (NYeC)	NY	www.nyehealth.org
HealthBridge Inc.	OH, KY, IN	www.healthbridge.org
Ohio Health Information Partnership (OHIP)	OH	http://ohiponline.org
Oklahoma Foundation for Medical Quality (OFMQ)	OK	www.ofmq.com
O-HITEC	OR	http://o-hitec.org
Quality Insights of Pennsylvania East	PA	www.qipa.org/pa
Quality Insights of Pennsylvania West	PA	www.qipa.org/pa
Ponce School of Medicine	PR	www.psm.edu
Rhode Island Quality Institute	RI	www.riqi.org
South Carolina Research Foundation	SC	www.healthsciencessc.org
South Dakota REC (SD-REC)	SD	www.cahit.dsu.edu
Qsource	TN	www.tnrec.org
North Texas REC	TX	www.dfwhc.org
West Texas HIT REC (WT-HITREC)	TX	www.ttuhsc.edu
CentrEast REC	TX	http://centreastrec.org
University of Texas Health Science Center at Houston	TX	www.shis.uth.tmc.edu
Health Insight	UT	www.healthinsight.org
VHQC (Virginia Health Quality Center)	VA	www.vhqc.org
Vermont IT Leaders	VT	www.vitl.net
WI-REC	WA	www.wirecqh.org
Wisconsin HIT Extension Center	WI	www.whitec.org
West Virginia Health Improvement	WV	www.wvhealthimprovement.org/wvhii/home.aspx

Hospitals and health systems

Office practices are in high demand. Although the past trend was for hospitals to purchase a practice, hospital systems are opting to create alignment through IT rather than through acquisition. Each patient that comes to his or her hospital or to your clinic for a procedure resulting in an admission helps the hospital's bottom line. Therefore, a local hospital may be willing to invest money and resources to help you implement an EHR and connect to their hospital.

Here's how your local hospital can help you:

- ✔ **Vendor selection and management:** Hospitals and health systems receive bulk purchase pricing for EHR software or hardware, have access to a larger budget than your practice, and go through a rigorous vendor selection and contracting process. You can benefit from their experience and may have an opportunity to participate in their vendor selection process or narrow your list of vendors because they've done the work for you. Check with your local health system to find whether they're issuing requests for information (RFIs) or conducting demonstrations of EHRs that community physicians can attend. You can also benefit from the health system or hospital's ability to manage the vendor, and set and maintain stringent performance benchmarks for both the technology and professional services, such as project management, system configuration, and training. Organizations need to ensure that the ambulatory EHR they select can integrate well with their hospital systems.

- ✔ **Facilities and training:** Until you're ready to implement, it's nice to have somewhere to go to look at the system and figure out what works best for your practice. Hospitals and health systems often set up training programs — with a training room — to make sure their providers have a good training environment. In addition to providing space, hospital systems often set up "test beds" with fake patients so that you can go through training that's more realistic.

- ✔ **Interface development and maintenance:** Hospitals and health systems generally have IT departments that are well versed in determining interface needs and working with vendors to ensure that the interfaces developed meet all requirements. When partnering with a hospital or health system, there's much incentive for the IT department to ensure their system supports your practice's workflow without interference. Also, you'll have someone nearby to call if you have any problems.

- ✔ **Customer support:** If you implement your local hospital's EHR, you're their EHR customer. Rather than calling an 800 number that routes you to who-knows-where or waiting for someone new to call you back every time, you get a live person. Your hospital wants your business, so there's incentive to provide you with good customer service, including access to readiness assessments and planning for your practice, training, and post–go-live support. Additionally, your practice physicians and staff will likely need onsite support when you first start using the system; this presents an opportunity for you to get to know some of the team you'll be working with for a long time.

Hospitals are prohibited by law from giving you an EHR and paying for all of the services associated with the implementation. However, a hospital can provide significant financial contributions for your implementation. Some hospitals may offer to pay up to 85 percent of the EHR software and implementation costs, and other health systems may just negotiate significant discounts from vendors that they can pass along to you. Also, because many independent physicians work with multiple hospitals, you can review the options from each hospital and make the best choice for you. Here are eight important questions to ask your hospital(s) when you are investigating EHR vendor options:

✔ Do you have a strategy to help implement EHRs for any non-employed physicians who work at your hospital?

✔ Have you already decided which vendors you will use?

✔ Is there more than one choice? (Many hospitals are working with two to three vendors.)

✔ What is the cost for each physician? (In other words, how much is the hospital paying?)

✔ Is my contract with the hospital or with the vendor?

✔ What ongoing support, if any, will the hospital provide for each clinic (training, IT, optimization)?

✔ What is the timing of the rollout and how do I "get in line"?

✔ How do I get involved?

Professional organizations

Professional organizations that serve both providers and staff offer help with EHR adoption. A wealth of information is available including specialized Web sites, magazines, newsletters, online discussion forums, and (we like this the most) access to your peers. Professional societies and organizations exist to support and help you. Most professional societies also have policy awareness, so they're tracking legislation, Meaningful Use criteria, and certification closely to provide you with what you need to know.

Check out these organizations for help with EHR adoption and information:

- ✔ **American Association of Family Physicians (AAFP; www.aafp.org):** AAFP knows that its entire membership is faced with implementing EHR and is a priority population under the HITECH Act. AAFP wants to help physicians get their incentive dollars, and overcome the reimbursement and financial challenges encountered by family physicians. AAFP proactively established the AAFP Center for Health Information Technology (www.centerforhit.org), a Web site with resources for physicians that also offers additional member-only resources, such as "Find a doctor like me" and a physician product reviewer/EHR user directory.

- ✔ **American College of Physicians (ACP; www.acponline.org):** Like the AAFP, the ACP is fairly progressive with respect to EHR adoption and development of resources to help its community. ACP established the Center for Practice Improvement and Innovation with a specific focus on Health Information Technology. This site also provides great resources and discussion forums. We like (sorry, members only again) the small practice discussion groups. ACP also helped create AmericanEHR Partners, a free Web site with resources and tools to implement EHRs (www.americanehr.com).

- ✔ **American Academy of Pediatrics (AAP; www.aap.org):** AAP's EHR-related resources are part of a larger Practice Management Online feature that includes *Implementing an Electronic Health Record Toolkit,* a module that helps prepare pediatric offices for the transition, vendor selection, implementation, and realization of EHR benefits and challenges. This tool offers the best pediatric practice management information, tools, and resources for pediatricians and their office staff in one easily accessible Web site.

- ✔ **American Medical Association (AMA; www.ama-assn.org):** The AMA is very involved in health IT policy circles as well, so its health IT Web site nicely organizes EHR and stimulus-related information. If you want to really dive into some of the policy aspects of the HITECH Act, check out the Stimulus 101, 102, and 103 compilation of frequently asked questions related to the stimulus. This site also has one of the niftiest Web sites we've seen so far with a U.S. map you can click to find the RECs in your state, complete with the services they offer and contact information.

- ✔ **National Association of Community Health Centers (NACHC; www.nachc.org):** The NACHC Web site includes EHR Selection Guidelines for health centers in selecting an EHR vendor developed by HRSA with participation from NACHC and several health center representatives.

  ✔ **Health Information Management and Systems Society (HIMSS; www. himss.org):** HIMSS is pretty much the biggest professional organization supporting the health IT community — including hospital/health systems and vendors. The HIMSS Web site is a wealth of information and a good starting point for in-depth resources related to what's going on in the industry. We particularly like its "Topics and Tools" section — a nice educational resource and glossary of terms and a good place to go when you're wondering about what some acronym means or you want to learn more about an area of health IT.

Quality organizations

While professional organizations mainly serve their specific members, many national organizations focus on improving the overall quality of health for everyone. You can turn to several quality organizations to find out more about meeting EHR-related standards of quality for care through electronic information sharing. Most of these organizations are broad-based in focus but include parameters for acceptable and encouraged use of electronic health records.

Check out these organizations:

  ✔ **Agency for Healthcare Research and Quality (www.ahrq.gov):** The AHRQ is the health services research division of HHS that focuses on the place of research within the healthcare industry, including research in quality improvement, patient outcomes, and clinical practice and technology assessment.

  ✔ **Ambulatory Care Quality Alliance (www.ambulatoryquality alliance.org):** The AQA is a wide-reaching group that includes several stakeholder groups who agree on ways to measure performance and report their findings to consumers to improve patient outcomes.

  ✔ **American Medical Association Physician Consortium for Performance Improvement (www.ama-assn.org):** The PCPI is an AMA-sponsored group committed to improving quality of care and patient safety. This group develops, tests, and maintains evidence-based clinical performance standards.

  ✔ **American Health Quality Association (www.ahqa.org):** The AHQA says its mission statement is an "educational, not-for-profit national membership association dedicated to promoting and facilitating fundamental change that improves the quality of health care in America." This association is an umbrella organization representing a national network of community-based quality improvement organizations (QIOs).

- ✔ **National Committee for Quality Assurance (`www.ncqa.org`):** NCQA is a private, 501(c)(3) not-for-profit organization dedicated to improving healthcare quality. You may be familiar with the NCQA seal, which designates that an organization is managed well and delivers the highest quality of care and service based on the mantra "Measure. Analyze. Improve. Repeat." One vital aspect of this designation is an organization's use of electronic information. Organizations must meet 60 standards and report their performance in more than 40 areas to receive the NCQA seal, many of which are IT-related. Additionally, NCQA developed the Health Effectiveness Data and Information Set (HEDIS) tool that gauges performance on key ambulatory healthcare measures.

- ✔ **National Guideline Clearinghouse (`www.guideline.gov`):** The NGC is a resource for the public so all stakeholder groups (patients in particular) can review evidence-based clinical practice guidelines.

- ✔ **National Quality Forum (`www.qualityforum.org`):** The NQF is another useful not-for-profit organization that seeks to create and implement a national strategy for quality measurement and reporting.

Understanding EHR Certification

The Office of the National Coordinator for Health Information Technology (ONC) has designated ONC Authorized Testing and Certification Bodies (ONC-ATCB). To keep it easy, we refer to ONC-ATCB certified products as "certified EHR" or "certified products." These bodies will conduct certification of EHRs to be included in ONC's Certified Health IT Product List (CHPL) in 2010. You have to be using a product that is on this list to qualify for incentive dollars. This means that EHR vendors are making key upgrades to their systems to ensure their compliance with the latest Meaningful Use criteria and newest certification requirements.

Starting in September 2010, ONC announced three ONC-ATCBs and indicated that it may continue to announce more organizations. See the current list of certification bodies at `http://healthIT.hhs.gov/ATCBs`.

The ONC-ATCB certification ensures that the product is capable of meeting ARRA/HITECH Act criteria but, as always, you must ensure that the product meets your needs. In addition to ARRA certification (AKA certification by an ONC-ATCB), other certification programs go beyond the criteria established by the federal government. Look at the certification programs described in the following sections to determine whether your practice should include the capabilities of each certification program.

CCHIT

The Certification Commission for Health Information Technology (CCHIT) is a not-for-profit group whose mission is to accelerate the adoption of health IT by improving quality, safety, efficiency, and access. A relatively new organization, CCHIT (founded in 2004) is largely in the business of providing certifications for EHRs (which it has done since 2006). CCHIT was the first organization in the industry to certify EHR functionality and interoperability, so it's not surprising that it is an ONC-ATCB as well as additional certification programs for EHRs.

Previous and CCHIT Certified 2011 criteria were developed through a voluntary, consensus-based process that takes the opinions of multiple stakeholders into account.

CCHIT offers two certification programs:

- ✔ **ONC-ATCB Certified 2011/2012 (www.cchit.org/products/onc-atcb):** This program certifies complete EHRs and EHR modules and is recognized by ONC to certify that an EHR meets ARRA certification criteria. Certification by this program translates to Medicare and Medicaid incentives.

- ✔ **CCHIT Certified 2011:** This independent certification (separate from the ONC-ATCB certification program) includes a thorough inspection of your EHR's integrated functionality, interoperability, and security. This certification offers an enhanced level of verification and validation of additional EHR capabilities to support varied and improved workflows, clinical decision support, and care delivery. This is CCHIT's next generation of programs geared at certifying complete EHR functionality. In this case, key aspects of successful use are verified at live sites, and usability is rated (ambulatory EHRs only).

- ✔ **Previous certification programs (www.cchit.org/previous_certs):** Prior to establishing the other programs, CCHIT offered many certification programs.

Drummond Group, Inc.

Drummond Group, Inc. (DGI) was founded in 1999 and has years of experience in testing services for auditing, quality assurance, conformance testing, test lab services, software certification, Web services testing, and interoperability testing. DGI has tested products in multiple industries "such as automotive, consumer product goods, healthcare, energy, financial services, government, petroleum, pharmaceutical and retail." DGI announced its first ONC-ATCB–certified EHRs on October 3, 2010. View products certified by DGI at www.drummondgroup.com/html-v2/ehr-companies.html.

InfoGard

InfoGard was founded to provide accredited IT security assurance services to customers worldwide. InfoGard has expanded its services in developing many certification programs, the latest being EHR certification. Find out more about InfoGard at www.infogard.com.

The role of standards and standards organizations

Every profession has standards, and the healthcare industry makes them a priority to ensure the health and safety of the American public. Now, with the dawn of the EHR age, those standards extend to the realm of health information technology as well. Luckily, some organizations' sole purpose is to set and monitor health information technology standards.

HIT Policy and Standards Committees

The HIT Policy Committee was created under the Federal Advisory Committee Act (FACA) as a result of ARRA to make recommendations to the National Coordinator for Health Information Technology (HIT) regarding development and adoption of a national health IT infrastructure (http://healthIT.hhs.gov/FACAs). In other words, the HIT Policy Committee works to help us all move toward a paperless health IT structure. The committee uses several workgroups to achieve its mission, including workgroups focused on

- ✔ Meaningful Use
- ✔ Certification and adoption
- ✔ Information exchange
- ✔ National Health Information Network (NHIN)
- ✔ Privacy and security
- ✔ Strategic planning

The HIT Standards Committee, which also comes to you courtesy of ARRA and FACA, is in charge of making recommendations to the National Coordinator for HIT about standards, implementation, and criteria for electronic exchange of information. The committee prioritizes policies developed by the policy committee, and employs the following workgroups:

✔ Clinical operations

✔ Clinical quality

✔ Privacy and security

✔ Implementation and adoption of standards

HL7

Health Level Seven International (HL7; www.hl7.org) is a not-for-profit organization that develops standards designed to create a framework for the use, exchange, sharing, and retrieval of electronic health information with the goal of supporting clinical practice management. The organization has more than 2300 members, including approximately 500 corporate members who make up more than 90 percent of all the information system vendors serving the healthcare sector. According to the organization's Web site, the mission of HL7 includes measures designed to

✔ Improve care delivery

✔ Optimize workflow

✔ Reduce ambiguity among stakeholders

✔ Enhance knowledge transfer among stakeholders

✔ Exhibit timeliness, scientific rigor, and technical expertise in processes without compromising transparency, accountability, or practicality

✔ Put stakeholders first

The Level Seven referred to in HL7 stands for the seventh level of the International Organization for Standardization (ISO) communications model for Open Systems Interconnection (OSI).

HITSP

The Healthcare Information Technology Standards Panel (HITSP; www.hitsp.org) works as a partnership between public and private healthcare sectors to create a set of standards that can enable operability among healthcare software applications. HITSP does this by supporting a local, regional, and health information network. Transparency is a big deal to the members of HITSP, and they work to maintain that open view into their processes by

- ✔ Opening membership to all interested parties
- ✔ Making work products available for public review and comment prior to approval
- ✔ Opening all meetings to membership participation

IHE

Integrating the Healthcare Enterprise (IHE; www.ihe.net) is an initiative created by healthcare professionals to improve the way computer systems in healthcare share information across applications, systems, stakeholders, and settings. IHE promotes the coordinated use of established standards, such as DICOM and HL7, to address specific clinical need in support of optimal patient care. Systems developed in accordance with IHE communicate with one another better, are easier to implement, and enable care providers to use information more effectively. Although IHE doesn't come up with new standards, the adoption of new standards to keep up with the demand of ever-changing clinical needs is encouraged. Think of the IHE as the friendly, neighborhood community officer who just wants everyone to get along and play by the health information technology rules.

NIST

The National Institute of Standards and Technology (NIST) is an agency of the U.S. Department of Commerce that is involved in several levels of healthcare IT interoperability and quality (http://healthcare.nist.gov). The institute works with major standards development organizations, professional associations, and the public to promote safe standards-based solutions for the exchange of healthcare information. NIST has been responsible for several initiatives and has a long-standing relationship with HHS and ONC, and is "responsible for leading the development of the core health IT testing infrastructure that will provide a scalable, multi-partner, automated, remote capability for current and future testing needs."

Now that ARRA is in effect, NIST has an even greater responsibility to promote the quality of healthcare information. NIST has developed test procedures for use by certification bodies (ONC-ATCBs). Specifically, as defined by ARRA and according to www.nist.gov/index.html, NIST aspires to

✔ Advance healthcare information enterprise integration through standards and testing

✔ Establish grants program for health enterprise integration centers

✔ Consult on updating the Federal Health IT Strategic Plan

✔ Consult on voluntary certification programs

✔ Consult on health IT implementation

✔ Provide pilot testing of standards and implementation specifications, as requested

Part II
Planning for an EHR

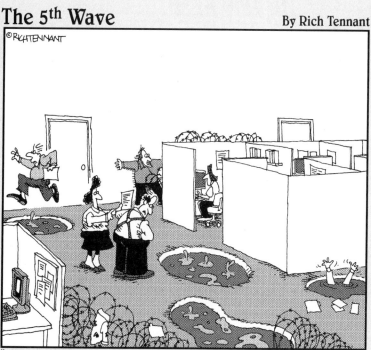

The 5th Wave   By Rich Tennant

"Okay, maybe a decent EHR initiative will improve our business performance, but I still think these sulphur pools and twines of barbed wire in the hallways are slowing us up in some ways."

In this part . . .

Bring on the meat of this book! Chapter 4 prepares you for the EHR readiness assessment to see whether the time is right for you to adopt a new system. Chapter 5 is where you play the numbers game, figuring the cost and return on your EHR investment. Chapter 6 gives you a tour of the vendor landscape and shows you what to look for in (and ask of) a potential EHR vendor. Chapter 7 covers the legal mumbo-jumbo that accompanies signing your vendor contract.

Chapter 4

Assessing Readiness

*W*hen you're ready to go vendor shopping, you can't just start making phone calls and writing checks. Take some time to find out whether your practice is truly ready to make the move to an EHR. You might think things would operate much smoother without all of that paper, but don't forget you have to preload and ultimately shred or store those files, train the staff, and evangelize the benefits of EHR to your patients. The moral of this story is to make sure you're ready.

Adoption and implementation processes are neither quick nor easy, so take the time to be absolutely 100 percent sure that you're ready to make the move to a paperless existence. Your successful move into an EHR-based way of life requires more than enthusiasm (you have that already). Your entire organization must be on board with the concept and resulting changes in procedure, workflow, and technology. A lack of readiness in those areas leaves your organization wide open for EHR adoption failure, which is something you don't want. Guarantee your paperless success by assessing your organizational, technological, and clinician readiness.

If you find that your organization is not ready in one category (say, organizational readiness), do not review potential vendors. Instead, make a list of what your priorities are in that particular area and dedicate some time to address those needs before moving forward with EHR adoption.

Gauging Organizational Readiness

First things first. Time to take the temperature of your organizational readiness. You need a strong idea of whether your overall organization is ready for EHR adoption and implementation.

This is the perfect time to revisit some of the reasons why you (or those who started your organization) are in the healthcare business. You have to think big picture and blue sky. Go back to the original business plan and see whether any of those hopes, fears, opportunities, and obstacles still rings true. Then think about how they jibe with your potential EHR initiative.

Developing a mission and vision

If you start with documents that you already have, like a business plan, then you have a jumping-off point for thinking about your future with an EHR. Think of this as an opportunity to re-vision your practice in terms of mission. Consider your overall organizational mission and values and how you want the EHR to enhance or improve them. Here are some initial big-picture questions to ask:

- What is your organizational structure?
- How do you define your organizational culture?
- What is the current structure of your leadership team?
- What are your strategic goals?
- How do your technology objectives align with your overall organizational goals?
- Can you apply EHR initiatives across the board? In other words, can you use EHR to improve your primary strategic areas?
- Do your leadership performance criteria match up with your organizational goals?
- How does staff performance affect your goals?

After you answer these questions (and any other ones you think up), you can begin to envision (or re-vision, as the case may be) your organization's mission and values. Think of these in simple terms, like this:

- **Vision:** What you hope to do.
- **Mission:** What you're going to do (action-oriented).
- **Values:** What's important to you. Organizational values can be about anything from how you conduct research or interact with patients and colleagues to issues of quality and conduct.

That's not so bad, right? Now, think about how an EHR can help you achieve those visions and missions and help you hold true to your organizational values. Ultimately, address how you want the paperless technology to reinforce the good work you're doing in your organization, improve the processes or workflows you want to change, and enhance the relationships among your organizational stakeholders.

Identifying goals for a specific EHR implementation

If you have some overall organizational goals, think about how EHR implementation fits into that picture and set some specific goals for the process. Believe it or not, you really do have to ask, "Why *are* we doing this?" The answers may seem obvious (eventually, you will have to use EHR, for example), but if you think about the question in terms of what outcomes you want, the answers provide much stronger clarity. We all do things because we have to from time to time, but doing them usually makes more sense when we focus on the benefits.

Then fit your organizational goals to your EHR goals. Take a second look at the values that you've identified and brainstorm EHR goals in light of them. You can create a simple matrix (using your favorite spreadsheet software) that joins organizational goals with EHR goals. See Table 4-1 for an example.

Table 4-1	Goal Matrix Example
Organizational Goal	*EHR Goal*
Communicate better with patients	Secure messaging, patient portal, and PHR features
Streamline intake process	Scan insurance info directly into records and print demographic info from EHR for verification
Have better knowledge of patient prescription issues	Access medication history electronically and implement drug interaction/allergy notifications
Create more opportunities for patient feedback	User-friendly interface to share with patients
Improve billing accuracy	Automated coding features
Recoup more reimbursements	Coding accuracy checks
Streamline prescription refills	Electronic prescribing features
Allow for more physician mobility	Off-site accessibility

(continued)

Table 4-1 *(continued)*

Organizational Goal	EHR Goal
Open more dialogue with off-site colleagues	Chat, e-mail, IM, and file-sharing features
Create patient education program	Downloadable brochures
Offer more flexible communication regarding appointments	Automated scheduling features and reminders
Share information more openly with Specialists or diagnosticians	Near real-time communication of lab results and radiology reports
Manage patient groups	Patient group management features

Determining a budget

Next on your to-do list is money management. Determining how to pay for an EHR (they don't fall off trees, remember?) plays a huge role in whether you proceed and how you proceed with EHR adoption and implementation.

Your budget should include more than just the sticker price of the EHR. Take into account costs associated with preparation, training, go-live, employee overtime, and added support.

We recommend including line items for the following:

- Hardware
- Software
- Chart conversion
- Training
- Installation
- Network connectivity
- Workflow redesign
- Loss of productivity
- Initial tech support
- Additional fees associated with training (travel expenses for offsite personnel or vendor reps, catering, and so on)
- Annual software maintenance, upgrades, and support

✔ Hardware upgrades or replacement

✔ Construction or facility fees (for example, adding permanent hardware or changing a file room to a patient exam room)

✔ Miscellaneous

You can read more about the specifics of EHR costs and budgeting in Chapter 5.

After you settle on a budget that works for your organization, you have to pay for all these EHR goodies. Thankfully, you have options, and you don't necessarily have to set aside a huge chunk of your annual organizational budget at one time:

✔ **Paying upfront:** This is exactly what it sounds like — you pay out your entire EHR budget. Obviously, you can't pay for ongoing costs (say you need to replace broken hardware two years down the road), but you can pay the majority of the year-one adoption and implementation costs directly to the vendor in one lump sum.

✔ **Deferred payment:** Many vendors offer a deferred payment plan. Think "installment loan" here. If you've ever bought a car via a special promotion (No money down! Pay only interest for 12 months!), then this will sound familiar. The good news is that it's often a wise choice if you can't shell out thousands of dollars in one shot, and the payment schedule is often based on the size of your practice. For example, you can get the "no money down" deals if you have a certain number of physicians or have been in business for a few years. You can also set up a few months' worth of deferred payments and slowly increase payment size over time, or structure a monthly payment system based on practice size. Be sure to ask your potential vendors about their options. Some RECs are working with banks to offer financing assistance, too.

✔ **Percentage of charges:** Similar to the deferred payment model, this option allows you to start your implementation with little or no money up front. Some vendors provide billing services for practices through their own company or one of their partners. Rather than charging you money up front, they take a percentage (generally, 5–8 percent) of your billing charges for their services. Also, many billing services have documented the ability to appropriately increase your billing and reduce your accounts receivable (AR), thus saving you more money.

In addition to paying for an EHR yourself, make sure to investigate the other sources of financial support that might exist, including hospital systems and regional extension centers. You can read more about these sources in Chapters 3 and 6.

Creating a realistic timeline

Knowing how you will roll out your new EHR is just as critical as knowing how you're going to pay for it. Like wedding planning (this is like a marriage, remember?), you need to have a master to-do list and a timeframe for executing the major steps leading to and following the day you start using your EHR (your *go-live date*).

State and federal milestones affect your ability to earn EHR incentives. Be sure you set up your EHR timeline to meet those important goals. See Chapter 5 for detailed information about incentive programs.

Start your timeline by considering what elements of your to-do list are time dependent. Think about how long each part of the process will take and plan for it. Generally, you should expect the following timeframes:

- ✔ **6–9 months prior to go-live:** This initial phase of EHR investigation is when you assess your needs, create an EHR wish list, research vendors, get employees on board, make a final vendor selection, and set training and go-live dates.

- ✔ **5–6 months prior to go-live:** The excitement builds as you name an EHR implementation team, identify needs based on an assessment of your practice, choose your vendor, and begin the cost-benefit analysis process, which you read about in Chapter 5.

- ✔ **3–4 months prior to go-live:** Consider this "ramp-up" time and think about EHR in terms of your available resources. Start to make decisions about transitioning from paper charts, install hardware, work with the vendor to customize your EHR, make initial preparations for training, and communicate to patients the changes.

- ✔ **1–2 months prior to go-live:** Training and testing. Time to work with the vendor on tweaking the software to fit your needs and to overcome any glitches you might see. Confirm that your new workflows (see Chapter 8) are incorporated into the software. This is also the time to prepare your staff for the training and go-live phases by creating a constant EHR dialogue (regular EHR meetings and updates are key) and to make sure staff knows to reduce patient flow in the coming weeks to account for training time. Most practices will start training 3–6 weeks prior to their go-live date, depending on the size of the practice, and then provide refresher courses right before go-live.

- ✔ **Go-live and 1 month following:** Breathe. Just breathe. In, out, in, out. Oh, and try to have some fun. Build your joke file ("An EHR and a paper record walk into a bar . . ."). You have increased staff and reduced patient load for the go-live and subsequent weeks. This first month is about just getting through — focusing on the patient and using the basic EHR functions.

✔ **1–3 months post go-live:** After using the EHR for a while, you start to take notice of what works and what doesn't. Share those experiences and ask for feedback from your staff (and colleagues outside the office) on how the EHR is working. Hosting regular debriefings to discuss questions, concerns, and new ideas is a great activity. Additionally, this is a good time for the vendor to provide some post go-live training for you and your staff to help reinforce good habits and point out some advanced functionality that you can start using now that you have the basics.

✔ **3–6 months post go-live:** After you're familiar with using the EHR and have received some retraining and advanced training, it's time to assess what's working and identify areas you want to improve. Reserving some of your training or implementation time to discuss this with your vendor is a good option, as is consulting with experienced peers or others that can offer optimization guidance.

This is just an example of how your EHR process might pan out. Remember that every practice is different and has varying needs, so the timeline should be based on your circumstances. For example, you may want to spend 1–2 months researching vendors before you commit and plan for go-live or reduce the timeline in half if you have an experienced staff and are ready for the change. Make your timeline fit your needs.

Figure 4-1 shows an EHR timeline.

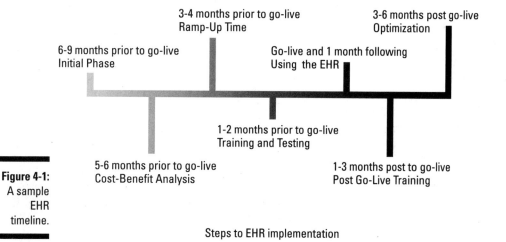

Figure 4-1:
A sample EHR timeline.

3-4 months prior to go-live
Ramp-Up Time

3-6 months post go-live
Optimization

6-9 months prior to go-live
Initial Phase

Go-live and 1 month following
Using the EHR

1-2 months prior to go-live
Training and Testing

5-6 months prior to go-live
Cost-Benefit Analysis

1-3 months post to go-live
Post Go-Live Training

Steps to EHR implementation

Building the team

Team building can identify key players to help facilitate your move to EHR. A strong leadership team is essential to ease the transition to an EHR while providing ample handholding for the rest of your organization. Two roles to fill here are

- ✔ **A physician champion:** If you are a one-doc operation, the choice is obvious. However, if you have multiple physicians in your practice, choose someone who can be enthusiastic and educated about what EHR can do for the staff. Generally, employees will follow suit if they see a physician who's confident about the switch to EHR.

- ✔ **A day-to-day leader:** Select an office manager who can coordinate everything from timelines and goals to nitty-gritty details, such as who brings the bagels for the training session.

If you are part of a large practice, consider having an EHR advisory board of stakeholders (someone from the front office, billing, nursing staff, and so on) that meets weekly or monthly to discuss how EHR is functioning.

After leadership is in place, think about whom else should be on your team. Here are some ideas:

- ✔ **A vendor rep:** Think of your vendor rep as a team member, not an adversary (or merely a sales rep). He or she is there to make sure the EHR adoption is going smoothly to keep you all working toward the same goal.

- ✔ **A representative from each office role:** Include a nurse, a medical assistant, a front desk staff member, and a billing staff member on the team. Essentially, you're looking for a champion for each role. They'll make decisions that affect everyone, so ensure they understand their new responsibilities and prepare them to be champions for their colleagues.

- ✔ **Outside resources:** If you're part of a larger organization, you may need extra support and expertise for your implementation. Your vendor rep may provide additional resources (for a fee) or recommendations for outside consulting help. Additionally, ask your friends and colleagues who have already implemented EHR for their recommendations, too.

Every employee is a part of this team, even if they are not directly involved with the finer transition details. Because you all have to rely on EHR in some capacity, keep everyone in the transition loop with ongoing communication and ask whether anyone has questions or concerns while you move through the process (they will). Also, be mindful of everyone's time commitments both in and out of the office. Work with your staff to set up times for training sessions on reduced patient load days.

Determining Technology and Infrastructure Readiness

After you assess everything from your budget and personnel to your mission statement and timeline, you can take stock of your technology situation. Evaluate your hardware resources, determine what you will need for the EHR, and pinpoint what sort of IT support you will need going forward.

Overall assessment of your technology and infrastructure readiness should include the following issues:

- ✔ Capability of the current IT infrastructure to support EHR
- ✔ Security requirements
- ✔ Existing systems
- ✔ New system needs
- ✔ Employee technology comfort levels
- ✔ Existing and future backup plans for data storage and restoration
- ✔ Ability or desire to host information in-house
- ✔ Dedicated or contracted IT staffing

In the following sections, we look at the major IT readiness assessment issues to see where your practice stands.

Evaluating current hardware

Start by assessing your current hardware. Work with your vendor rep to make a list of your hardware that works with the new EHR software. The vendor can and should provide you with a list of requirements for software, network connectivity, and hardware needs. Additionally, the vendor may help provide the hardware to you or point you toward a preferred resource that can help.

Don't be afraid to ask for help because technology can be one of the more daunting aspects of the EHR experience. Talk to your friends and colleagues at other practices, reach out to your local hospital for advice or support, and ask the vendor to connect you to other successful practices to get their input and advice.

If you find that you need to discard some good working hardware, consider offering a sale to another practice and put the money into your EHR war chest. Cha-ching!

You should analyze the functionality and condition of the following:

- Servers (if hosting onsite)
- Desktop workstations
- Laptops and tablets
- Fax machine
- Scanners
- Voice recognition equipment
- Handheld devices (such as PDAs or smartphones)

List the pros and cons for any hardware that falls into the "questionable" category. If, for example, you have a slightly outdated scanner or fax machine that syncs with the new software without problems, determine whether keeping it (initial savings) outweighs chucking it (saves you from buying a new scanner two years down the road).

Determining new needs for hardware devices

Your EHR hardware wish list probably contains items to make EHR as usable as possible in any setting, from the front office or exam room to the break room or physician's car. You want hardware that adequately suits your mobility needs and your workflow and functionality needs. To that end, ask whether you want to go for flashy or functional. If you go with flashy (say that gorgeous touchscreen tablet), remember that you may sacrifice some functionality (oops, you can't touch that gorgeous touchscreen tablet after the kid in room 4 yakked all over the place and you). We're not saying that flashy can't be functional; we're saying temper the temptation of flash with a touch of functional.

Many hardware decisions are based on the limitations of your office setting. For example, if your exam rooms are very small and you have to move in and out of them quickly, maybe a more mobile option like a laptop or tablet is the way to go instead of a desktop or rolling cart workstation. Think about your ability to connect to a wireless network, too. If your office is in an office building made of cinderblocks, chances are you might have a tough time getting a signal without standing near a window. Therefore, choose hardware that can help you overcome that issue.

Where you locate office computers in the front office and other work areas (like the nurses' station) depends on how you use the space, too. If, for example, two employees work in the front office, choose hardware that will help them maintain their own space yet access commonly used equipment (like a scanner). In other words, if the office space is shared, maybe you shouldn't opt for the big screen and clunky CPU tower.

Additionally, think about the patient while you consider your hardware options. You want to keep your patients engaged throughout their visit, and they may not find staring at your back the entire time the most enjoyable experience. If you choose a workstation option, make sure you can converse with the patient while using the system and turn the monitor to show patients different components of their record, such as radiology films or trends of their cholesterol numbers.

That's a lot to keep in mind, but luckily, hardware categories are simple to remember:

- ✔ **Server:** If you are hosting your EHR onsite, you have to have a server capable of holding all the patient record information. This doesn't apply if you're implementing an ASP/SaaS EHR. All the computers in your office communicate with the server to get the needed information. Choose a server large enough to handle your patient record load while your practice grows that offers enhanced backup and security features.

- ✔ **Workstation:** If you want the practice's computers to stay in one place, you want workstations, and you decide where to position them. Many practices set workstations in the main traffic areas of the practice (front office, nurses' station, billing office, and exam rooms) so that you can access one and enter your information while you pass by. This option may be expensive because you have to buy a lot of hardware, but a good option for large offices or settings that may be too hazardous for toting around a tablet (such as an ER).

- ✔ **Wireless tablet:** This is a really fun toy. If you have a smaller practice or a very tech-savvy group of folks, you will likely want to go with the ultimate in mobility — the tablet PC, which weighs only around three pounds. This device allows you to use a stylus to write notes onto a screen that then transfer into the health record. This is an economical option because you have to supply only one tablet per provider in the office that each can carry from room to room. However, if you go with this option, physicians have to learn how to use the EHR and the tablet. Some staff members may find writing with a stylus a challenge, especially if they tend to use their own version of shorthand that only they understand.

- ✔ **Laptop PC:** You have a bit of both worlds with a laptop PC. A laptop can be stationary thanks to a docking station and mobile so providers can take it from room to room. However, it does weigh about twice as much as the tablet PC.

- ✔ **Handheld PDA:** This is the tiny version of a tablet. Most handheld PCs now have touchscreen capability, so you use them as you would a full-size tablet. However, if you don't want to see things in an incredibly tiny font, a handheld device probably isn't for you. However, PDAs are super mobile, can fit in your pocket, and travel well. More and more EHR vendors are providing iPad, iPhone, and other smartphone applications that are great for reviewing patient information on the go or out of the office.

- ✔ **Scanner:** You can go with a flatbed or a sheet-fed scanner, similar in look and feel to a fax machine. Sheet-fed scanners work just fine, but if you want the ability to scan smaller documents without having to fish them from the depths of the machine, a flatbed scanner might be your best option. Some scanners also offer an add-on device especially for scanning small items, such as insurance cards.

- ✔ **Patient kiosk:** An emerging trend in practices is to place limited functionality workstations or kiosks in patient waiting areas and check-in areas. These kiosks allow patients to check in, pay bills, and review or update their demographic information.

Your vendor rep is an excellent resource when making hardware decisions for your new EHR, as are colleagues who have already made the move. Consult your vendor or professional society for a list of peers using the same system. Ask them what works for them, what is most efficient, and what they would do differently if they could have a hardware do-over.

Deciding to host locally or remotely

Now you're ready to think about hosting. Not a party (though one probably sounds good right about now), but your EHR. You have two choices: local hosting or remote hosting.

Local hosting means that you house the server that maintains the EHR information right there in your office. To make this work for you, you have to budget for not only the server but also the tech support that goes with maintaining the server and any networking components and computer workstations that access the server. The onus to secure, maintain, and manage the server is on you, the local host.

Remote hosting, generally called an application service provider (ASP) or software as a service (SaaS), is a great option if you don't want the cost of server hardware. In this case, the software lives on a secure offsite server, you provide the individual workstations and any necessary networking, and pay for high-speed Internet access. Additionally, you pay the hosting company for its services.

Several major differences exist between a locally hosted EHR and a remotely hosted system. By reviewing these differences, you can determine the best fit for you and your practice.

Locally hosted solution

If you have a practice with an IT staff and have strong feelings about controlling everything about your system and data, you should consider the locally hosted model.

Characteristics of a locally hosted solution include the following:

- ✔ Hardware and software are located at your practice.

- ✔ Your practice is responsible for all maintenance and support of the hardware and software. Either an onsite staff or a contracted company supports your needs.

- ✔ No Internet connection is required to access patient and practice data — the EHR runs on your internal network.

- ✔ Your EHR vendor may supply software configuration support including ongoing training and optimization.

- ✔ Your practice pays larger upfront costs but reduces long-term expenses to just small monthly maintenance fees.

ASP/SaaS or remotely hosted model

Generally, the ASP model involves relinquishing some control and responsibility of the data, the software, and some of the hardware. Also, payment options and cost may be significantly different for an ASP than locally hosted EHR. With ASP, you essentially lease the software and continue to pay a larger monthly fee while you use the system.

Key ASP characteristics include the following:

- ✔ Hardware and software are located at a remote location.

- ✔ Someone else is responsible for the care and maintenance of the hardware and software.

- ✔ Internet connectivity is required to access the software.

- ✔ All users access the system through a Web browser or application on their device.

- ✔ Your practice makes monthly lease payments for the life of the system.

Getting connected to network reliability

If you decide to have the vendor or some other third party host your EHR software, you have to use your network's Internet connection to reach your patient's information. Therefore, if your Internet connection goes down, you can't get the patient information you need. If you're in a location with shoddy network reliability, a remote hosting model is probably not for you.

Additionally, discuss backing up your information with the vendor. Some vendors can provide an onsite terminal that houses patient information that can still be accessed even if the Internet stops working.

IT staffing

Regardless of what type of hosting you choose, you need some help in the IT department, if for no other reason than to assist you with maintenance and repair of your workstations, scanners, or fancy tablets. If you don't already have a technology support service, start shopping for one. Your vendor rep should have some suggestions, and an IT specialist may be available as part of your EHR package. Be sure to check with your rep for more information. Also, see if your local hospital is willing to help support you in this area.

Though your IT representative may not have all the answers to your tech questions, he or she should have the ability to seek out and report those answers to you.

Evaluating Clinician and Staff Readiness

When you have an idea of your technical readiness, think in detail about clinician and staff readiness, particularly in terms of culture and technical knowledge. The sooner you know how ready your staff and physicians are for EHR, the quicker you can move forward with implementing the goals and benchmarks detailed in your timeline.

Culture

Consider how your practice's corporate culture may affect your readiness for the EHR move. Practice culture, in this case, deals with how the people in your organization interact with one another and how they will respond to adopting and implementing EHR.

Leadership

Take into consideration your leadership team's readiness to juggle multiple EHR-related tasks, such as information management, financial considerations, human resources, and technical concerns. Not every physician in your office needs to be an expert in all things EHR-related; that wouldn't leave them much time for what they do best — patient care. However, your physicians should be ready to assist in what may be the biggest corporate transition your practice ever sees.

Find out whether anyone in your practice has experience leading a large-scale change initiative. If you're lucky enough to have someone like this on staff, enlist him or her to your leadership team ASAP.

Staff

Obviously, your office staff is on your readiness checklist. These stakeholders most likely have to access multiple portions of the EHR frequently. Therefore, get an idea of how they feel about this significant change to their routines and workflows. Sometimes, one of the biggest issues with EHR transition is the reluctance of employees to embrace new technology and processes. Barriers during the transition process can result in resistance against

- ✔ Practice leadership
- ✔ Transition team members
- ✔ Number of changes
- ✔ Frequency of changes
- ✔ Organizational changes from converting to EHR
- ✔ Technology itself
- ✔ Office staff who are succeeding with EHR

Many causes for EHR resistance are rooted in good, old-fashioned fear of the unknown. Causes for staff resistance to EHR may include

- ✔ Learning a new skill set
- ✔ Scrapping old habits and processes
- ✔ Feeling incompetent in front of coworkers and practice leadership
- ✔ Fear of being replaced by a machine
- ✔ Pressure to improve performance
- ✔ Pressure to make fewer mistakes now that everything is automated
- ✔ Fear of software failure

Don't let your employees' EHR fears get you down. Having concerns is perfectly normal because EHR changes how staff members perform their jobs. The key is to find a way to overcome those fears and move on to assess your team's ability to work together to make this transition happen. Consider these questions when assessing staff readiness, but you'll likely come up with your own, too:

- ✔ How can you get employees comfortable with change?
- ✔ Are your team members committed to the effort?

- Can employees work as teams? If they already do, how?

- Are clinicians ready to use data and patient information to change the way they practice?

- Are employees familiar with the practice's mission, goals, and values?

- How much do employees know about EHR?

- Do employees think EHR adoption is imminent and just a matter of time?

- How willing are employees to perform the tasks associated with the transition (assessments, training, go-live, and so on)?

- What is the staff's confidence level in practice leadership's ability to implement EHR successfully?

Be sure to assess your organizational readiness based on how decisions are made and who makes them. Consider keeping an ongoing list of EHR transition responsibilities that you can tweak based on what you find in your readiness assessment.

Computer and technical skills

Assessing how people feel and what you think each will do once you implement your EHR is well and good, but very little of that matters if you aren't aware of the participants' computer and technical skills. Not everyone in the office has to be as savvy as Bill Gates, but they should have a basic technical skill set.

When creating your technical assessment, find out whether anyone has EHR experience from a previous clinical setting, medical school, or residence training. If so, great! These individuals can ramp up fairly quickly and, most likely, already speak the EHR language. If you find no one has any EHR experience, no worries. You might have some initial conceptual and terminology issues to work through, however.

General Internet experience is a plus. These days, you'll be hard-pressed to find anyone who hasn't at least used the Internet to look up information or send e-mail. However, a Luddite or two may be floating around here and there; therefore, find out the level of Internet experience each potential EHR user already has. If, for example, they have ever purchased anything from a Web site, they are probably familiar with basic security issues, buttons, how to point and click, and wait times for information downloads. If users are familiar with online maps, they probably know how to use Web-based visual references. If they know how to use a social network, they will probably take to EHR communication features like a duck to water. Examining clinicians' awareness of these everyday Internet tasks will give you a clue to how well they will make the move to EHR.

Considering typing skills, too, may not seem obvious, but many people in (and thriving in) the professional world are not proficient typists. Because the majority of day-to-day workflows involve a keyboard, typing proficiency is a big issue. Several good, free online assessment tools measure typing skills, so find one that works best for your team. After you find out how familiar staff members are with their QWERTYs, you can take action to improve their typing skills.

Check out `www.typingtest.com/games` and `www.goodtyping.com` for quick training solutions.

Conducting assessments

When conducting readiness assessments, you have a wealth of options. Your potential vendor reps can recommend some useful assessment tools, and you can go online and search for them. You have two options here: a formal EHR assessment tool or a self-created survey based on the EHR goals you identify earlier in the process.

Several formal assessment tools are available, and some EHR companies create personalized versions that you can use at little or no charge. Most formal assessment tools are matrix format so you can view several aspects of readiness at one time. You then assign a number (say 1 for "not ready" and 5 for "ready") to each category and/or subcategory, such as leadership, culture, organization, strategy, technical skills, training, accountability, patient involvement, budget, and so on. Here are a few formal survey tools that you can access online:

- ✔ AmericanEHR Partners practice readiness assessment at `www.americanehr.com`

- ✔ California Community Clinics EHR Assessment and Readiness Starter Assessment. Visit `www.nachc.org/client/EHR_Starter_Assessment_final.pdf`

- ✔ The Info-Tech Research Group Templates & Policies Center EMR Readiness Assessment Questionnaire. Visit `http://archive.healthit.ahrq.gov/portal/server.pt/gateway/PTARGS_0_890628_0_0_18/EMR%20Readiness%20Assessment%20Questionnaire.pdf`

- ✔ Regional Extension Center Web sites

Figure 4-2 shows the EHR readiness assessment tool offered by AmericanEHR Partners. We recommend looking at a few readiness assessment tools and picking one that seems to address areas of concern in your practice. Typing *"EHR Readiness Assessment"* into Google yields quite a few options.

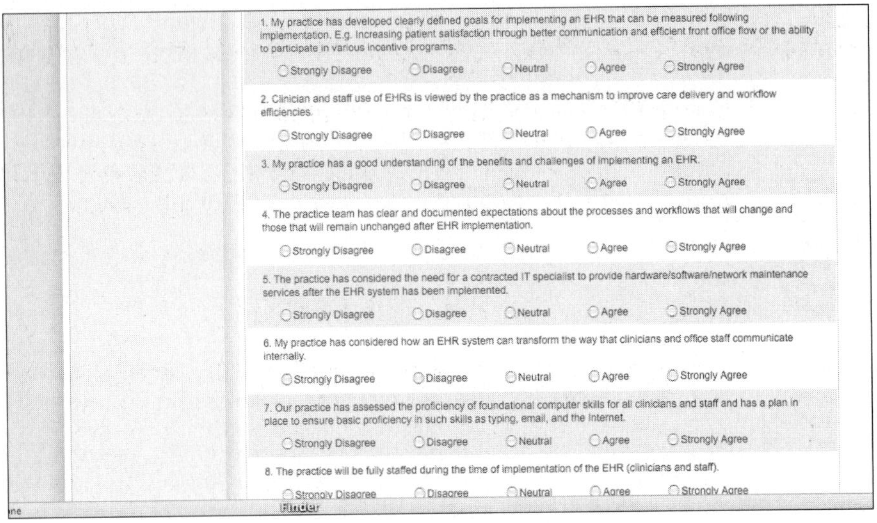

Figure 4-2:
American-
EHR
Partners
readiness
assessment.

You can also conduct paper-based or online surveys that you create and customize based on your EHR research. Several free online survey tools include

- ✔ Surveymonkey.com
- ✔ Wufoo.com
- ✔ Polldaddy.com
- ✔ Kwiksurveys.com
- ✔ Tigersurvey.com
- ✔ Zoomerang.com
- ✔ Questionform.com
- ✔ Freeonlinesurveys.com

Whether you're assessing the EHR readiness of your practice's physicians, staff, or patients, you have options and can create assessment criteria that address your specific organizational mission, values, and goals. The key to assessment success is to communicate your findings, build enthusiasm for how EHR can help staff achieve their professional and personal goals, and involve everyone in the process so each person knows what to expect at go-live.

Knowing What to Do if You're Not Ready

In your EHR journey, as in life, you might find that you're just not ready to move on. Say you complete the EHR readiness assessment and think, "Uh . . . I'm not certain we can do this right now." Relax. Take a big cleansing breath. Here's what to do if you have to leave your EHR initiative at the altar.

It's okay to not be ready

Give yourself permission to *not* be ready for EHR. Really! The point of doing all of this assessing is to see whether this huge change in your office culture and day-to-day workflow makes sense for you and your staff.

Though moving to EHR is in your future (you do want that incentive money, after all), it doesn't have to be your immediate future. This is where your assessment results come in very handy. Review them, make lists of areas where physicians and staff may fall a bit short in the readiness department, and then use those findings to map your EHR plan. Moving to a paperless world will happen — maybe just not today.

Determining initiative importance

Deciding an EHR initiative is a no-go can be good news. How can that be good news, you ask? Because you're being honest with yourself and not committing thousands of dollars to an initiative for which you might be woefully unprepared. Trust us; your investors (and you) will thank you. Additionally, by declaring your practice not ready, you create an opportunity to sharpen your EHR focus, decide what you want from the process most, and set a timeframe that best suits your needs. This is your chance to improve processes and skills in anticipation of your EHR initiative, no matter how far down the road.

Use your assessment findings to decide how important the EHR initiative and individual aspects of it are to your practice. If, for example, you see that your employees are experiencing a great deal of trouble with coding and billing issues, thus affecting your bottom line, you know that you need a solution sooner rather than later. However, if processes are to everyone's satisfaction and you're moving to EHR because doing so is inevitable, perhaps you hold off until the timing is right. Determine how your EHR goals jibe with your team's readiness and prioritize your EHR implementation based on that. Perhaps you'll find that you can, for example, ramp up technical skills quickly or discuss global organizational issues in the background to make EHR a high priority. Determine EHR's importance to you and solidify a timeframe that offers you the most benefit.

Getting your staff ready

When you decide on an EHR timeframe — even a long-term process — get your staff on board and let them know how the transition schedule will affect them.

Though EHR implementation may be two or three years away, make it a part of your office conversation and keep staff informed at regular meetings. Address some of the readiness issues you discover during assessment, and get them creating a working environment that complements EHR. Prioritize any action items, remedies, and next steps that result from the readiness assessment and ask staff to participate in finding useful solutions. If, for example, you see that your decision-making processes could use some clarification, consider that a high order concern (HOC) and dialogue about how everyone can streamline decision making. Or, if half of your office uses the "hunt-and-peck" method of typing, perhaps everyone can agree typing proficiency is a low order concern (LOC). In that case, work together to ramp up typing training but make it fun — host a typing training session with prizes, catered lunch, and an early stop time.

The key word here is *together*. This is your opportunity to create a stronger team, so get everyone invested in the improvements you need to make before moving to EHR.

Chapter 5

Determining the Cost, Benefits, and ROI

You already know that you're going to have to shell out the big bucks for your new EHR, but just knowing the cost of your hardware and software isn't enough to provide you with a clear picture of the true cost of the initiative. To really know how much the EHR is costing you, you have to consider the basic costs in conjunction with other factors, such as costs that may occur down the road and potential benefits. You're not doing this EHR thing because it's fun (but we hope one day, it will be); EHR is about realizing clinical, financial, and operational benefits.

In this chapter, we show you how to create a detailed budget based on EHR costs, benefits, and *return on investment (ROI)* — the size of what you get in light of what you spend. (ROI also refers to *release of information*, but for the purposes of this chapter, we're talking about your return on investment.) Calculating the cost is the last part of determining your EHR readiness. After all, how can you be ready if you don't know what the EHR will cost you or the benefits you'll achieve?

ROI factors items that aren't easy to quantify, benefits such as improved documentation and patient satisfaction, the effect of changed roles and responsibilities, and downtime caused by the implementation process. In other words, ROI provides you with the truest picture of your EHR costs.

So, get your calculator out and crunch the numbers, starting with system costs. And no, you can't claim that we said there would be no math!

Centers for Medicare & Medicaid Services (CMS) estimates that the average cost for an eligible professional to adopt a certified EHR is $54,000 per physician. CMS also estimates that the annual maintenance costs average $10,000 per physician. The cost is even higher for hospitals, which pay between $1 million and $5 million for installation; and $1 million annually for maintenance, training, and software upgrades.

Figuring Out the System Costs

The first thing on your cost list is the price you will pay for the EHR system itself. You probably know by now that this doesn't work in quite the same way as trekking down to your local office supply store to buy the latest version of Microsoft Office. You have several moving parts when it comes to system costs, so it's easiest to think of them in four categories: software and licenses, implementation and training, hardware and network infrastructure, and maintenance and support. Figure 5-1 shows how you can break down these costs.

Vendor reps have seen it all, so there probably isn't any request you can make that will shock them. Be honest about your needs, goals, and financial barriers. If they want your business, they will find a way to work within your budget.

Software

What you pay to license and use the actual EHR software is the bulk of your system cost. Most EHR vendors offer a software licensing price based on the size of your practice. If you have two physicians in-house, for example, a vendor will simply multiply the software licensing cost by a factor of 2. Much larger settings, like hospitals, would be charged a rate based on other factors because charging by physician could be challenging (most physicians don't actually work for the hospital; instead, they have privileges to practice in that setting).

Initial software costs vary widely based on vendor, but you can count on spending in the neighborhood of $2,000 to $40,000 per provider, depending on what kind of bells and whistles you add. Add-ons add up and increase your final software cost, so be sure to read more about them in Chapter 7.

Consider add-on software for such tasks as voice recognition as well, which add to your overall software costs. Most vendors do not provide this service as part of their offering, and you have to use third-party software, such as Dragon Naturally Speaking.

	Practice Hosted	ASP/SaaS Model
SOFTWARE AND LICENSES		
Physician licenses	$10,000 per provider	$500 per month
Mid-level licenses	$8,000 per license	$450 per month
Staff licenses	$5,000 per license	$250 per month
HIE Interface	$1,000 per license	$100 per month
Lab Interfaces	$3,000 per interface	$3,000 per interface
Patient Portal	$1,000 per provider	$75 per provider/month
IMPLEMENTATION AND TRAINING		
Training	$1,000 per day	$1,000 per day
Post Go-live Training	$1,000 per day	$1,000 per day
Go-live Support	$1,000 per day	$1,000 per day
HARDWARE AND NETWORK		
Laptop or Tablet Computer	$2,000 per provider	$2,000 per provider
Desktop Computer for Office Staff	$1,000 per individual	$1,000 per individual
Network Printer	$500	$500
High Speed Scanner	$900	$900
Server	$5,000	Not Applicable
Broadband Internet Service	$75/month	$75/month
Wireless Network	$1,000	$1,000
MAINTENANCE AND SUPPORT		
Software Maintenance	18% of software fees per year	Not Applicable
Back-up and Storage	$1,000 per year	Not Applicable

Figure 5-1:
An example cost benefit analysis.

Implementation costs

The hard work you do in anticipation of the EHR transition is time and money well spent. Though you may not envision the tasks you, your team, and the vendor are doing as actual dollars spent — you didn't write a check for them — they are, and you should account for them in your cost structure. Some vendors charge for implementation and project management; others bundle a set amount of services as part of a software as a service (SaaS) offering. Additionally, you may choose to use outside consultants to support your implementation.

Plan to spend roughly $75–$150 per hour on implementation costs, with an average implementation time per provider of 35 hours, which includes customization, training, and network setup.

Here is a detailed look at implementation costs:

- ✔ **Initial planning and procurement:** These are the costs involved with conducting readiness assessments, researching potential vendors, creating a timeline, and narrowing your list of potential vendors. You will find that many of these tasks take a toll on your time, which has a dollar value, so it's not always simple to estimate how much these things cost. You read more about people costs later in the chapter.

- ✔ **Contract negotiation:** Back and forth, back and forth. That's how contract negotiations work. You spend quite a bit of time working with your future vendor to establish parameters for how your relationship will work. Costs here may include travel expenses, legal oversight — make sure your lawyer triple-checks that contract — and your time.

- ✔ **Data migration:** This is what you've been waiting for — moving all of those cumbersome paper files to an electronic environment. But it doesn't happen by magic. Someone has to physically scan those files and input information into the new system, which — you guessed it — costs money.

- ✔ **Installation:** You may pay the vendor a flat rate for installation services, which will include multiple visits from the vendor rep and any ancillary IT support staff who get your system up and running. For small practices (usually fewer than five providers), many vendors are doing a 100 percent remote implementation (after the contract is signed, the vendor completes the system design and training and support from their headquarters, not at your office). Be knowledgeable about the level of support you're getting and what it's costing you.

✔ **Customization:** If you require customization beyond what's typical or what the vendor offers, you may need to pay separately for custom implementation services. Such services provide you access to a business analyst or application specialist who can determine your requirements and implement those changes into the EHR.

✔ **Workflow redesign:** Like system customization, this is often an add-on service. Vendors generally have predefined established EHR-enabled workflows that might work for your office. Or your practice may require a lot of assistance to make the transition to these or other optimized workflows. This service generally requires a clinical or implementation specialist or consultant to work onsite at your practice and is almost never included in the base price of an EHR.

✔ **Training:** Training is also a part of your implementation cost. Most vendors include some level of training in your overall package cost, and you can always negotiate for more. Training costs may vary based on the training type. In-house training sessions from the vendor rep may cost more than, say, a series of webinars that your staff can access online at their leisure. Be sure to push for the type of training options you want during the contract negotiation phase. We talk more about different training options in Chapter 11.

Ongoing maintenance and support

When your EHR is up and running, you have to keep it healthy. The software has to be maintained with updates, quality checks, and security add-ons. Software and hardware, like new cars, can become obsolete as soon as they are developed — someone is always designing new technology. Chances are your vendor will continue to update software systems based on such factors as emerging technologies and ever-changing legislation.

You also want the support of your vendor rep to make sure that your practice's questions are answered and your team members can use the software to full capacity. You will likely pay a fee for year-to-year vendor/tech support, with the typical annual fee running close to 18 percent of your software costs for an EHR that you are hosting at your practice. In an ASP/SaaS model, both licensing and ongoing support costs are built into your monthly fees.

Many EHR vendors include a year or two of software maintenance and support in the upfront system cost as an incentive, so be sure to ask your rep if that is possible. At a minimum, make sure that you're not paying for upgrades within the first two years of implementation or for Meaningful Use capabilities.

An introduction to ROI and developing a benefits framework

Before venturing into a purchase, you have to know your return on investment (ROI) to prove that your brand new EHR is really worth the software it's written on. ROI quantifies and communicates your costs and benefits to help you set the approach, measurement, and monitoring categories for a benefits framework.

You already know that transitioning to the EHR is going to save you time and money over the long term and improve patient care. The key, though, is to understand what the EHR is going to do to your bottom line in the near term. Your practice is a business and it has to be sustainable, financially speaking. Think of ROI as you would a picture. Everyone can take your word that the Grand Canyon is a thing of awe-inspiring beauty, but seeing a picture really drives your point home. ROI does just this — it paints an accurate picture in financial terms of the benefit your EHR provides.

That said, financial ROI isn't the primary method for deeming your EHR efforts a smashing success or a raging failure. Most medical professionals would agree that ROI is a secondary objective meant to help you visualize and improve operational goals (which are paramount in terms of benefit). Benefits and your ROI can be qualitative as well as quantitative. In other words, if you can prove you are getting a solid return on your investment, you can prove that you are improving in measurable ways as a result of EHR implementation. The trick is to accurately determine what constitutes success in each category you define. Therefore, when creating your list of EHR goals (see Chapter 4), include performance indicators that you can easily track and quantify.

To prepare employees and physicians to realize the highest ROI, make sure you (or someone else on the transition team) has a firm grasp of what it costs to deliver care and, as a result, selects the best system for your practice needs. Most importantly, ensure that all stakeholders are on board with the change and provide them with the tools they need to succeed during the transition, including paying for additional training or simply offering additional pep talks. And, of course, be sure to have a plan for setting goals for and tracking your ROI as part of your benefits framework. You can

- Create the costs and benefits framework prior to EHR implementation
- Encourage stakeholders to help decide ROI criteria
- Determine meaningful metrics
- Establish a process for keeping track of ROI data
- Capture data
- Track ROI throughout the timeline established in your cost-benefit analysis

Determining Infrastructure and Hardware Costs

Your shiny new EHR system will probably need some shiny new hardware. When you conduct your readiness assessments, you should assess your hardware needs in terms of what you already have that works, what you have that won't support a new EHR system, and what you need to add to your hardware mix. (See Chapter 4 if you still have to assess your hardware needs.)

Here are some cost considerations associated with EHR-related hardware:

- ✔ **Facility upgrades:** If you have to add desks, put in a wireless network, or reconfigure exam rooms, account for such costs under this category. For example, if you are going to convert the old chart room to a billing office, you will need to add the cost of construction, networking, new furniture, adding phone lines, and so on.

- ✔ **Servers:** Your hardware costs depend on what sort of hosting scenario you choose. If you want to host the system in-house, meaning that your practice stores the EHR data on a server in your office, you have to purchase a server and the peripherals that help it work. If, however, you plan to use a SaaS or ASP hosting model, in which your data is stored on a server located offsite, then this cost does not apply. Servers typically cost around $5,000, but that depends on the number of providers that are supported by your server.

- ✔ **Desktop workstations:** You may already have some desktop workstations that will "talk" to your new EHR software. If so, good for you because that means lower hardware costs! However, you may find that even if you have some existing, useful hardware, you may need to add more workstations to account for the increased number of staff members who will need to access EHR. For example, perhaps your medical assistant (MA) used to enter patient vitals into a paper record, and that was his or her only record-related function. Now that you've gone paperless, your MA has to enter that info into a computer, so he or she will need to access the EHR at a workstation of some kind.

    You can purchase workstations for decent prices, especially if you're buying multiple units. Costs can run about $2,000. Ask your vendor for purchasing recommendations.

- ✔ **Laptops and tablets:** If you're going mobile, you need the right gear. Serving the same function as a desktop workstation, a laptop or tablet allows you to work while you move throughout the office. Understandably, these devices cost more than traditional workstations, and you can expect to pay from $2,000 to $4,000.

- ✔ **Fax machine:** Most EHRs include online fax capabilities that eliminate traditional faxing hardware. However, there will be times when you need to send something over the old phone line. If your fax machine doesn't work with the new EHR, count on purchasing a new one for approximately $200 to $400.

- ✔ **Scanners:** Your scanner will become your new best friend. You'll use the scanner to preload paper charts into the new EHR. Additionally, you'll scan driver's licenses and insurance cards. EHR-capable scanners run close to $1,000.

✔ **Kiosks:** Some practices are installing kiosks in their waiting rooms to encourage patients to complete some administrative and data entry tasks before they come into an exam room. For example, patients could enter some of their medical history and lists of medications.

✔ **Handheld devices (such as PDAs or smartphones):** These are really fun toys. Check with your vendor rep to see what brands of smartphones and PDAs work best with EHR software to review patient information or maybe even place orders. Most mobile companies will cut you a corporate deal if you order multiple units, so shop around for the best price on devices and monthly plans.

If the numbers for your EHR wish list scare you, take heart. You can get creative and find some ways to cut costs without cutting quality. For example, you don't have to use just one kind of workstation. Consider opting for mobile tablets for the provider and a few workstations for employees. Mixing it up could save you a bit on the bottom line. Or perhaps you can hang on to the older scanner or fax machine that works just fine with the new EHR software. You might also ask your vendor rep whether leasing equipment would save you any money in the long run.

Considering Sweat Equity: People Costs

While a lot of costs associated with your EHR transition seem pretty obvious (such as your software cost), some expenses are a bit more complex. Take, for example, the people costs your practice will incur to adopt and implement EHR. People costs are related to the labor (both vendor reps and IT professionals) involved with the implementation and the in-house cost of time spent training and ramping up for the go-live.

Expect your vendor and IT professionals to charge between $75 and $150 per hour. Clinical professionals or consultants with significant experience in EHR run even more — double these rates. You can ask potential vendors to estimate hours spent working with your practice to implement EHR and train the staff to have a ballpark figure when you run the numbers.

The complex people cost, however, comes during implementation, training, and go-live. If, when you conducted your readiness assessments, you found that a lot of labor involved pulling charts, running back and forth to the fax machine, and looking for lost information, you'll be thrilled to know that EHR will reduce those costs. But in the short term, you will lose valuable time spent ramping up for go-live and getting back to normal afterward. Trust us, EHR is worth it in the long run, but it's vital that you account for these hidden costs to realize a more accurate ROI.

Here are a few people costs you can expect during implementation, training, and go-live:

✓ **Training:** You're going to spend some "people dollars" during the training phase. Because no "real" work is done when an employee is sitting in the conference room or watching a webinar, you need to account for those instances per employee. (It's not like your employees will agree to not being paid for their training time.) To calculate your people cost for training, figure time spent multiplied by hourly wage. For example: 10 hours of training per employee x $25 per hour x 5 employees = $1250. The cost you pay a trainer is often included in the overall package the vendor sells. But if you decrease your patient load to accommodate training schedules, there's a cost associated with decreased revenue for that period, too. On average, you should plan to reduce patient load by at least 25-50 percent during the first week of go-live.

✓ **Overtraining:** You can have too much of a good thing, and you will pay for it if you go overboard with the training. Refer to your readiness assessment to determine roughly how much training your staff needs. If, for example, everyone in the office can type 90 words per minute, you probably don't need to waste time training them to type. Gauge how your employees are responding to the training and add on more training if you deem it necessary.

✓ **Too little training:** Don't let the vendor rep convince you that his EHR is easy to understand. No matter how user-friendly your new EHR appears, it's a complex animal, and you need to participate in adequate training to use it properly. If you undertrain, you run the risk of losing time post go-live because no one knows what they're doing, and you'll have to request further training. Also, if you're not effectively using the EHR, you run the risk of increasing medical errors and putting your patients at risk rather than improving their care. Work with your vendor rep to schedule adequate training and have a plan B in case you need more work in a particular area. Schedule some retraining to occur after your practice begins using the EHR, too. Therefore, save a little bit of your training allocation or budget for post go-live when everyone understands most clearly how to use the EHR.

✓ **Workforce adjustment:** You may need to add or eliminate staff positions when you move to the EHR. Perhaps you'll host your information in-house and want a full-time IT specialist. Or maybe you'll eliminate a transcriptionist position because the EHR essentially removes that need. Though you'll be saving money by not paying a salary, you will have costs associated with letting that person go in the form of final severance, vacation time payout, and insurance costs you wish to provide.

✓ **Transition team time:** Whether your transition team is a one-man or one-woman operation (that is, you) or a team of multiple stakeholders, you need to account for time spent doing EHR-related activities outside your primary job description. Run the equation just as you did to figure training costs.

It's called go-live, not go-perfect. Give yourself (and your employees) a break — the EHR is a product designed by humans, for humans. Just go with it.

✔ **Additional employee meetings:** Keeping employees informed about the EHR transition can be a challenge, so keep those communication lines wide open. You might have to extend staff meetings by a few minutes or schedule meetings specifically to cover EHR topics. If so, account for these times in your people costs.

✔ **Eliminating paper charts:** Shred baby, shred! Preloading all that chart information and discarding those paper charts will feel good, but they aren't going to scan and shred themselves. Someone in your office has to take time from her scheduled work to do it. You have options here. You can assign a few team members a few hours to work on this project, offer incentives to come in on weekends or other off-hours, or even hire a student or temp to do the scanning and shredding as short-term gig. Any way you go, though, it's going to cost you some hours in the labor department.

You can get as detailed as you wish when figuring people costs, so if you really want to account for the 20 minutes it took for you to grab sandwiches for the transition team lunch, go for it. The more accurately you capture your people costs, the more accurate your ROI will be.

Affording employees the time to research vendors, head a transition team, or even participate in training is a challenge (some might say it's close to impossible). The truth is you cannot skimp on these areas. Dedicate the appropriate level of participation to the process to make the EHR work in the long run.

Tracking Potential Benefits

Benefits . . . that's what you've been waiting to see. You may feel as if you just completely emptied the practice's bank account, but — surprise! — you will recoup some of those costs. Many EHR benefits will pay you back over the long term. From the obvious plusses, such as the ability to pull charts anytime and anywhere, to the less obvious benefits, such as improved stakeholder satisfaction, the benefits are practically unlimited.

You will measure benefits in a variety of ways, and it's important to realize that some ROI measures will have a hard dollar amount associated with their achievement, and others may be tougher to quantify.

Categorizing key EHR benefits

When you create your spreadsheet that lists your EHR costs and benefits, add categories in the Benefits section. Developing your benefits framework helps your stakeholders see where your benefits reside so they can better visualize how an EHR can help your practice. Here are a few categories of long-term EHR benefits that can serve as a framework for monitoring and measurement:

- ✔ **Patient safety and quality:** Improved decision making, access to records, overall quality, overall patient safety, reduced errors, firm clinical guidelines and decision support, and increased information sharing.

- ✔ **Financial benefits:** Improved charge capture and documentation, reduced transcription costs and staff expenses, increased patient volume and profit, improved collection rates, decreased claim denials because of coding errors, elimination of transcription costs, and expanded office space.

- ✔ **Efficiency and operations:** Improved workflows and prescribing methods, decreased charting time, improved patient scheduling efficiency, short turnaround time for insurance claims and lab results, increased access to patient information, and less time spent returning calls.

- ✔ **Stakeholder satisfaction:** Increased and improved customer service, decreased patient wait time, greater employee retention, and more patient interaction time.

The best benefit, hands-down, is universal chart access. Physicians, employees, outside specialists, pharmacists, and diagnosticians can (with the proper access) pull charts any hour of the day from any location. You'll be surprised to find how much time you spent dealing with paper charts, and the time saved translates to a monetary benefit.

Suppose that a physician sees, on average, 100 patients a week, and each chart pull takes approximately five minutes. That's 500 minutes a week the physician (and other employees) could spend providing more care or performing other duties. Now, multiply those 500 minutes by the pay rate of the employee who handles those charts — maybe $15 an hour for a front office staffer, $10 an hour for a transcriptionist, and a whole lot more for the physician. We're talking cash money back in your pocket.

You can also account for chart pull time in terms of quick reference items not related to a regular visit, such as checking on a prescription, changing patient contact information, or returning a patient phone call. Every minute you no longer have to spend pulling a paper chart is another minute of time in the benefit column.

According to Partners HealthCare, creating a new paper chart costs approximately $2, and physically pulling a paper chart costs $5 each time. Cha-ching.

The EHR's effect in the billing department is another big benefit. An improvement in coding can realize a cost benefit of thousands of dollars per year. Not only does an EHR help you work faster; you improve coding and charge capture accuracy, which means you experience a higher return of approved insurance claim payments. Partners HealthCare found a 1.5–5 percent increase in overall billing because of improved charge capture. Not too shabby.

You can list many other EHR benefits in your final analysis depending on how detailed you want to be with the price of the payoffs. Check out this list of EHR advantages (and feel free to add more of your own!):

✔ **Patient safety and quality measures**

- Reduced medication errors because of drug/drug, drug/allergy and other interaction checking

- Reduced duplicate testing

- Dose checking

- Improved adherence to quality guidelines, such as immunizations or cancer screenings. (If you're part of a PQRI program, then this will mean increased financial returns, too.)

- Improved medication management through electronic prescribing

✔ **Financial benefits**

- Reduced or eliminated transcription costs

- FTE reductions or improved utilization

- Supply savings

- Improved efficiency leading to increased productivity

- Improved coding and charge capture

- Decreased denials

- Reduced form costs

- Improved cash flow through faster claims submission and payment

- Reduced chart handling costs

✔ **Efficiency and operational benefits**

- Less time spent dealing with prescription management

- Better office visit workflow efficiency

- Quicker lab and radiology turnaround

- Improved scheduling of office visits

- Improved referral processing including authorization, scheduling and preparation

✔ **Stakeholder satisfaction**

- Higher employee satisfaction

- Stronger employee retention

- Increased patient access to personal medical information

- Lower patient wait times
- Increased engagement of your patients in their own care
- More time for patient care
- Quicker patient communication via e-mail and instant messaging

Some of these measures are easier to quantify than others, allowing you to factor their contribution more accurately into your overall return on investment. But, just because you can't financially quantify something doesn't mean it has no value.

Factoring in the incentive payments and penalties

Thousands of clinics implemented EHRs before there were nice federal incentive packages, but fortunately, you can use both traditional ROI metrics and the additional ARRA stimulus funding to offset your costs. If you're eligible for incentives, they play a huge role in your analysis of costs and benefits. Remember that you will only receive the CMS financial incentives after you become a "meaningful user" of the EHR and meet each specific requirement.

How much you can potentially receive depends on the year you begin qualifying. Here is the payment breakdown:

- ✔ If your first qualifying year is 2011 or 2012, you can receive up to $18,000 in EHR-related incentives.

- ✔ If you don't apply until 2013, the annual incentive payment limits in the first through fourth years are $15,000, $12,000, $8000, and $4000, respectively, for a total of $39,000.

- ✔ The maximum amount of incentive payments you can receive under Medicare is $44,000. That's not chump change.

- ✔ If you meet the Medicaid patient volume requirements, you can receive a higher potential first year payment, which is an incentive payment of $21,250 and a total of $63,750. Your timing to receive this payment is limited by your state's level of readiness to process Medicaid payments for Meaningful Use, so it will be important to check with your specific state's Medicaid office or REC to obtain this information.

The EHR incentive rule suggests a 90-day reporting period for the first year you apply for and receive an incentive payment. The rule proposes an EHR reporting period of an entire year for every year thereafter. Keep that in mind while you move through the reporting process.

Tables 5-1 and 5-2 show how the incentives and potential reductions are expected to work from 2011–2017.

Table 5-1	Medicare Incentive Payment Schedule	
First Payment Year	**First Payment Year Amount, and Subsequent Payment Amounts in Following Years**	**Reduction in Fee Schedule for Non-Adoption/Use**
2011	$18k, $12k, $8k, $4k, and $2k	$0
2012	$18k, $12k, $8k, $4k, and $2k	$0
2013	$15k, $12k, $8k, and $4k	$0
2014	$12k ,$8k, and $4k	$0
2015	$0	–1% of Medicare fee schedule
2016	$0	–2% of Medicare fee schedule
2017 and thereafter	$0	–3% of Medicare fee schedule

Table 5-2	Medicaid Incentive Payment Schedule	
First Payment Year	**First Payment Year Amount, and Subsequent Payment Amounts in Following Years**	**Reduction in Fee Schedule for Non-Adoption/Use**
2011	$21,250, $8.5k, $8.5k, $8.5k, and $8.5k	$0
2012	$21,250, $8.5k, $8.5k, $8.5k, and $8.5k	$0
2013	$21,250, $8.5k, $8.5k, $8.5k, and $8.5k	$0
2014	$21,250, $8.5k, $8.5k, $8.5k, and $8.5k	$0
2015	$21,250, $8.5k, $8.5k, $8.5k, and $8.5k	$0
2016	$21,250, $8.5k, $8.5k, $8.5k, and $8.5k	$0
2017 and thereafter	$0	$0

Source: CMS

Incentives are great, you say, but how will they really affect your practice? Will you actually get any of this money? According to CMS, you will. The CMS reports that they anticipate paying $14 billion to $27 billion in EHR-related incentive payments to eligible Medicare and Medicaid providers over the span of 10 years. These numbers do include room for adjustment for providers who do not achieve Meaningful Use by 2015 (approximately $2.3 billion to $5.1 billion), but that is still a lot of cash to be had for those who do comply. In addition to monetary gains are incentives that you can't deposit directly. By adopting and implementing an EHR, you'll net dollar savings at least equal to the initial cost you pay for the EHR (think of it as breaking even), and you'll contribute to the well-being of society's healthcare, which will result in billions of dollars' worth of savings over time. Not a bad deal for going paperless.

Participating in other incentive programs

It pays to report — literally. By participating in quality reporting functions, you can participate in incentive programs. For some reason, the government and healthcare industry want you to report on things. Who knew they liked reports? All kidding aside, it benefits you to report on quality, even beyond the scope of improving your office functions and patient care.

Pay-for-performance (P4P) programs were created by healthcare payers to encourage physicians to follow evidence-based guidelines for preventive and chronic disease care measures. In 2006, a *New England Journal of Medicine* article reported that more than half the health maintenance organizations (HMOs), representing more than 80 percent of enrolled patients, used pay-for-performance in their provider contracts. We're sure that number is much greater today, representing physicians who serve more than 150 million patients. According to a white paper published by EHR vendor Sage, P4P payments represent more than 7 percent of physicians' total compensation. Although that's not necessarily big bucks, every source of income counts. Would you walk away from a 7 percent raise?

Health Affairs (May 2010) published findings from a RAND Corporation study that found pay-for-performance programs might have an unintended consequence of lower payments for practices that serve vulnerable populations. This study also found that these practices have room for performance improvement, which is where the EHR and quality reporting can help.

Thanks to the 2006 Tax Relief and Health Care Act, the Physician Quality Reporting Initiative (PQRI) affects all physicians and eligible professionals who do business with Medicare. Think of it as the government's P4P incentive program. It's voluntary, but by reporting quality data on measures determined by the CMS, you can earn extra cash for your practice. You won't be a millionaire (practices average $630 a year), but it's more money than you had yesterday. Hey, it all spends.

Let's do the numbers: A breakdown of incentives

Hang on to your calculators. It could be a bumpy ride. Figuring out how, exactly, the EHR-related incentives work can be a daunting process. The many numbers and requirements can be a challenge to keep track of and difficult to apply to your practice. Consider this a little crib sheet to help you:

✔ Physicians (non-hospital–based) are eligible for Medicare incentive payments based on an amount equal to 75 percent of the allowed Medicare Part B charges, up to a maximum of $18,000 for early adopters whose first payment year is 2011 or 2012.

✔ Incentive payments would be reduced in subsequent payment years, eventually phasing out in 2016.

✔ Physicians who do not adopt/use an EHR system before 2015 will face a reduction in their Medicare fee schedule of –1% in 2015, –2% in 2016, and –3% in 2017 and beyond. The Secretary of HHS has the authority to make exceptions to this reduction on a case-by-case basis for physicians who demonstrate significant hardship (say a physician who practices in rural areas without sufficient Internet access).

✔ Physicians who report using an EHR system that is also capable of e-prescribing will no longer be eligible for the e-prescribing bonuses established by the Medicare Improvements for Patients and Providers Act (MIPPA); they will be eligible for HIT incentives only to avoid "double-dipping." Also, e-prescribing penalties sunset after 2014, so no physician will be subject to penalties for failing to both e-prescribe and use an EHR.

✔ Incentives under the Medicaid program are also available for physicians, hospitals, federally-qualified health centers, rural health clinics, and other providers. However, physicians cannot take advantage of the incentive payment programs under both the Medicare and Medicaid programs.

✔ Eligible pediatricians (non-hospital–based), with at least 20 percent Medicaid patient volume, could receive up to $42,500.

✔ Other physicians (non-hospital–based), with at least 30 percent Medicaid patient volume, could receive up to $63,750 over a six year period.

✔ In the event that the Secretary of HHS finds the proportion of healthcare providers who are meaningful users of EHRs is less than 75 percent, the Secretary is authorized to increase penalties beginning in 2018, but penalties cannot exceed –5%.

Source: American Medical Association's Explanation of HIT Provisions

Calculating Your ROI

After you determine your costs and benefits, you can accurately budget and plan for the entire implementation. You'll have a much easier time determining your actual and potential costs if you review vendor RFI responses and look at specific hardware costs early on. Estimating the financial (and other) benefits of the EHR prior to your implementation is more challenging but important. Achieving a true ROI takes time and, although the federal incentive structure may change some of this, you shouldn't expect the cash to start rolling in as soon as you turn on the EHR.

Follow the mantra "you can't measure what you don't monitor" before, during, and after your EHR implementation. For example, if you don't know how much you're spending on transcription, how will you know how much you're saving after you stop using the service? If you've never officially measured employee satisfaction, how will you know whether it improves or worsens after you go-live?

The process of monitoring the costs and benefits of your EHR continues throughout implementation and use. Stay vigilant in your measurement and tracking but not overwhelmed. Follow these steps to start the process and then work with your vendor and other support resources to continue.

1. **Focus on costs first. Write down each of these items:**

   - Each cost category (such as hardware, software, forms).

   - Each expense item.

   - An educated estimate of actual cost over a year (such as forms and transcription costs for a year).

   - Total all estimated costs.

   - Assign an owner from the practice to document actual costs after go-live.

2. **Identify key expected benefits:**

   - Write down each benefit category and subcategory.

   - Document appropriate national/industry benchmarks.

   - Document any current baseline measurements from your practice (such as percentage of established patients for each E&M code or current employee satisfaction scores).

   - Determine if specific information needs to be documented in the EHR to support a specific benefit metric.

   - Design the EHR and associated reports to support your benefit strategy.

   - Incorporate all of these benefit goals into your training and support materials.

3. **Track and monitor your progress:**

   - Create a schedule for running key reports from the EHR to measure your progress.

   - Review the output with appropriate operational owners and potentially all staff.

   - Make adjustments to the system, specific workflows, or training to optimize the EHR and your practice.

   - On a regular basis (quarterly or biannually), post your progress and calculate benefits and costs to determine your ROI.

Chapter 6

Selecting Your Vendor Partner

Choosing your EHR vendor is one of the first and most important choices you will make as part of this process. Before you dive into a detailed workflow evaluation and before you encourage your staff to participate in training, you have to pick a vendor and EHR product.

For ambulatory practices, implementing EHR technology is as close to marriage as it gets — you're partners with the technology until death do you part. Well, maybe not that long, but finding and working with a vendor who will be a great partner is critical. Much like finding a mate, the process takes time. Depending on the size of your practice or number of clinics in your organization, the vendor selection process can take some focused time.

The selection process may seem daunting when you think about all the steps involved, but if you follow a structured approach, you can select the right EHR for your clinic and engage your entire staff in the process.

Creating a Plan of Attack

Before you review Web sites with vendor information and start shopping for a partner, develop a plan and schedule that outlines each task in the selection process. Exercising a little discipline while you carefully think through each major step and requirement will save you both time and money. Whether you're the owner of the EHR plan or you're an employee who is helping in the vendor selection process, creating a game plan ensures that the primary decision-makers have all the tools they need to be successful. (And maybe you can suggest they read this book, too.) The first step in creating that winning game plan is determining the players on your vendor selection team.

Picking a team

Every team needs a captain, starting team members, and key people to come off the bench and provide a little extra help. The process of choosing your vendor is really no different, and a team approach allows everyone to have the opportunity to participate and appropriately share his or her thoughts and concerns.

Your vendor selection team should represent the perspectives of all stakeholders or at least all stakeholder groups in your office. We outline the team members from your practice in Chapter 4: a successful EHR implementation requires that the front office staff, the administrators, nurses, and physicians can effectively use the EHR. Therefore, they each need a role in the selection.

After you have a strong representation of office constituents (and even before hosting your first vendor selection meeting), be sure that you do the following:

- ✓ **Set expectations for the entire team and clearly define each person's role in the vendor selection process.** They need to know what you want each of them to provide in the vendor selection process and what sort of commitment is involved with the process.

- ✓ **Provide time on everyone's schedule to participate.** If you're involving other physicians (and you should), then give them the schedule relief to attend the meetings and demonstrations.

   Your fellow team members have day jobs. Whether they're employees of your office or physicians or staff stakeholders from elsewhere, they still have to perform their day-to-day functions in addition to helping you choose an EHR. So, cut 'em some slack if they can't make every meeting. Try to hold a few meetings before or after clinic hours, or during lunch where you offer some incentives such as food.

- ✓ **Value their participation and give their voice appropriate weight.** For example, if you feel that the front office staff will have the most interaction with specific features of the EHR, you might weigh their opinions on those features more strongly than those of other team members. If you think enough of them to be a part of the team, then it makes sense that their vote in the process should have some importance, too.

Refining your decision-making process

When you have your team in place, pinpoint who will incorporate the perspectives and opinions of the selection committee members and make the final vendor selection decision. You may want to have the only and final say in the selection, which may simplify the process but leave you open to criticism if employees experience problems later and the negativity that the decision didn't take into account staff needs and preferences.

Involve the influential people from your practice in the process even if they're not thrilled with the idea of using a computer to document patient care. In fact, get those naysayers engaged early so that you have ample time to address their concerns. When you get them on your side, their voices will provide invaluable support. Sometimes your harshest critics can become your most fervent supporters.

You can use several approaches to govern how you select a vendor. Review these three strategies to determine which one works best for your office culture and overall style of leadership.

Democratic

You can make decisions as a democracy and allow all participants to have an equal vote in the selection process. Here are the upsides:

- ✔ Everyone feels involved and has less room to complain about the decision.
- ✔ The perspectives of every stakeholder group are included in the selection process; therefore, the chosen vendor is more likely to suit all end users.

Here are the downsides:

- ✔ Everyone may not understand all the complexities involved in making the final the decision.
- ✔ You have a practice to run and if you involve everyone equally in the entire process, your overall clinic productivity may suffer.
- ✔ Including everyone equally takes time that may affect your overall timeline.

Benevolent dictator

You can run the process like a benevolent dictatorship and make the final decision on your own. Although you can involve others in the process, the ultimate decision and only vote is yours. Take the needs and hopes of each group into account and choose the vendor that best fits the needs of the entire practice. Here are the pros of rolling Queen Elizabeth style:

- ✔ This may be a quicker decision-making process and there is less likelihood that your timeline will be adversely affected.
- ✔ You understand all aspects of the decision, including any long-term implications.

And, the cons:

- ✔ If the vendor doesn't work out or you run into problems with software, it's your fault.
- ✔ Although the overall decision process may be shorter, the tax on your own professional time will be significant. Do you really have the time to do everything on your own?

Compromise

You can always compromise (most clinics do) between a complete democracy and a benevolent dictatorship. Involve many, possibly all, office members in at least part of the process by kicking off and presenting the plan to everyone. Then, communicate regularly, including progress updates, and let everyone participate in the vendor demonstrations. You can also involve a couple of representatives in the vendor site visits to increase involvement. Weigh the votes appropriately and allow for you, the captain, and a few key team members to share the primary responsibility of the final EHR choice. Here are the pros and cons:

- Pro: You get a balance of involvement and streamlined decision making.
- Pro: You can get every stakeholder group involved in both the process and decision-making, but add more weight to the practice leaders' votes.
- Con: Takes longer than deciding on your own.

Working within your timeline

Factor in enough time to conduct a thorough selection process and ultimately choose the best vendor product for you and your practice. If you have a specific (or approximate) go-live date, then work backward from that time. Here's a timeline you can work from:

- Account for one to two months for the initial work of researching, planning, and requesting information from potential vendors.
- Plan for one to two months of demo time, in which you meet with prospective vendors so they can demonstrate the capabilities and functionality of their systems.
- Allow for roughly one month to negotiate and make your final vendor selection.

You're looking at an approximate six month commitment, depending on how much daily time you wish to dedicate to the vendor selection process.

Documenting a plan

Put everything on paper, in a spreadsheet, or at the very least in a detailed memo to your team and staff. You don't have to use a fancy program to make a useful record of your plan, but if you're a multimodal kind of person, jazz it up with multiple platforms. Create recurring reminders, make a PowerPoint or Prezi plan that is interactive and colorful, or just make a useful Excel sheet that is easy to read.

Regardless of how you document your plan, include some goals, timeframes, and milestones by which you can chart your progress. Include a listing of set regular meetings and make note of required participation for your selection committee. The more specifics you can include, the more time you will save later by reducing the number of questions you will need to field from your committee.

Understanding the Vendor Landscape

Currently, there are more than 400 ambulatory electronic health record systems. That's right, 400! Some have been around for more than 20 years and many have come to life in the fertile soil of new health IT opportunities. Some have been developed by large technology superpowers and others have been created in the garages or home offices of physicians. The good news is that many of the vendor systems will work great for you and your practice, and that takes a little pressure off you feeling like you have to make the perfect choice.

Products bells and whistles vary, and many products cater to a specific practice size or specialty. Thus, it is important to develop your own requirements so you can find an appropriate EHR fit for you and your team. In other words, know yourself before you start looking for your partner. If you still need to access your needs, see Chapter 4.

With so many vendors, starting your search can feel overwhelming. The products in Table 6-1 cover a large majority of practices in the United States.

Look at vendors that are ONC-ATCB–certified and consider whether additional certifications such as CCHIT are important to you. At the time of this writing, the ONC-ATCB program had only recently launched, so check http://onc-chpl.force.com/ehrcert for the Certified Health Products List (CHPL) that meet Meaningful Use criteria and qualify for CMS EHR incentives.

Table 6-1	EHR Vendor Products	
Vendor	**Web Site**	**Product(s)**
Abel Medical Software Inc.	www.abelmedicalsoftware.com	ABELMed EHR
Allscripts	www.allscripts.com	MyWay, Professional, PeakPractice, Enterprise
Amazing Charts	www.amazingcharts.com	Amazing Charts EHR
American Medical Software	www.americanmedical.com	Electronic Patient Chart

(continued)

Table 6-1 *(continued)*

Vendor	Web Site	Product(s)
athenahealth	www.athenahealth.com	athenaClinicals
Cerner	www.cerner.com	PowerWorks
eClinical Works	www.eclinica works.com	eClinical Works 8.0
Epic	www.epic.com	EpicCare EMR
e-MDs	www.e-mds.com	e-MDs Solution Series
GE Healthcare	www.gehealthcare.com	Centricity EMR
Greenway Medical Technologies	www.greenway medical.com	Primesuite
Henry Schein Medical Systems	www.micromd.com	MicroMD EMR
Ingenix	www.ingenix	Care Tracker
McKesson	www.mckesson.com	Horizon Ambulatory Care
MDLand	www.mdland.com	iClinic EMR
MED3000, Inc.	www.med3000.com	InteGreat EHR
NextGen Healthcare Informatics Systems, Inc.	www.nextgen.com	NextGen Ambulatory EMR
Noteworthy Medical Systems, Inc.	www.noteworthyms.com	NetPractice EHR, NetPractice EHRweb
Pulse Systems, Inc	www.pulseinc.com	2011 Pulse Complete EHR
Sage Software Healthcare, Inc.	www.sagehealth.com	Intergy EHR

To know thyself (and thy practice), do a little reconnaissance and see which EHR vendors other practices are using and why. Snoop around, ask questions, and keep a running list of characteristics you hope to find in a vendor partner. Try these tactics:

- Talk with your specialty society to see whether it has tools to narrow your choices or whether it can provide an EHR recommendation or two.

- Check with the hospitals in your area to see whether they are supporting an EHR or planning their own implementation.

- Discuss options with your local colleagues to see which EHR they are using, how they like it, and how they made their choice.

- Use an online tool (available free or for purchase).

We list all the resources you could possibly need to narrow your vendor choices in Chapter 3.

Functionality is not the differentiator. How the vendor supports its client base, its responsiveness to issues and opportunities, and its ability to continually update and optimize its product sets apart the elite from the also rans. So don't base all your decision on the pretty demos vendors show you — get to the topics of training, support, and partnership.

With so many vendors in the marketplace, many companies either will fold or be acquired. Inquire about the vendor's viability in this competitive healthcare landscape. Ask the vendor, or conduct your own reconnaissance, for the following information:

- How long has the vendor been in business?
- How many practices does it support?
- Are there any plans for merging or being acquired by another vendor? (You likely won't get a straight answer, but it's worth asking.)
- How many sales in the last 12 months? What percentage of growth is that? Is it getting bigger?
- What's the average length of time its staff has been with the company?

You want (and need) this relationship to be a partnership between you and the vendor, so ensure your partner is going to be around.

Evaluating Your Technical Needs

The process of exploring your technical needs for the EHR and your practice can be a little daunting, but it is doable. Focus on what questions to ask and gather necessary information from the vendor and other sources.

Ask for help. If you are involved with your local hospital, its IT department may provide some helpful advice. Also, reach out to your local lab and pharmacies for their input.

Break down the topic of technology and focus on a few key questions:

- Where is the equipment and data stored? How often is the data backed up? Do you want local hosting or remote hosting? We help you evaluate what kind of hosting most benefits your practice in Chapter 4.

✔ How will you connect to outside information sources, such as labs, pharmacies, and hospitals? Evaluate how each vendor will support you and your clinic in sharing clinical information with other providers in the most efficient and secure ways.

✔ What equipment should you and your staff use?

Your patients receive care from many physicians, hospitals, pharmacies, labs, and care organizations. The EHR offers a way to connect you and your patients to those healthcare entities. Evaluate how each vendor will support you and your clinic in sharing clinical information with other providers in the most efficient and secure ways.

Make sure the EHR you select allows you to do the following:

✔ Expedite the referral process with another physician.

✔ Improve the admission of a patient to the local hospital.

✔ Provide the necessary information from a patient's recent ER visit or hospital stay.

✔ Send specific information directly to patients in a secure format to enable them to participate in their own care.

✔ Connect to the entire healthcare community through an HIE.

EHR facilitates sharing information in a multitude of ways, and most physicians use all four of the following techniques. Be sure to ask whether the vendor offers the following:

✔ **Integration between applications from the vendor.** For example, if you are using both the clinical EHR and the practice management (PM) system from the same company, patient information is stored and passed in the same program and does not require a separate interface to allow sharing.

✔ **An interface allowing two systems to talk to each other to share information.** An interface must be built, which requires both technical expertise and money.

✔ **Electronic distribution through e-mail or auto-faxing.** Many systems permit a user to send information to an outside entity provided that the other provider's information is stored within the EHR.

✔ **Print reports from your EHR that can be mailed or faxed to other care providers.** This method is not as technically sophisticated as the other three, but is very important in terms of practicality.

If you're purchasing the same PM system as your EHR, you still need interfaces between your clinic and the outside world. Generally, your contract addresses interface costs and the responsibilities of you, the vendor, and other entities, such as an outside lab company. Many 2011 Meaningful Use criteria require the

EHR to transmit or exchange information with other organizations; the amount of information to be exchanged outside the practice to meet 2013 and 2015 criteria will continue to increase. Some of this information exchange may be accomplished via integration with your local, regional, or state health information exchange (HIE). Consider asking these questions of each potential vendor during the request for information (RFI) and interview processes:

- ✔ Do you have experience interfacing with our PM system?

- ✔ Do you have experience interfacing with the EHR system that our local hospital uses?

- ✔ What are the costs for each type of interface? How much is covered in the contract? Are there additional maintenance costs for the interfaces?

- ✔ What happens when one of the outside system upgrades and the interface needs to be changed? Who does the work? Are there extra costs for our clinic?

- ✔ What happens when our EHR upgrades and EHR interfaces need to be changed? Who does the work? Are there extra costs for our clinic?

- ✔ Are costs for the e-prescribing module included in the vendor contract?

- ✔ Are you participating with a local or regional HIE, and is there any associated cost for the clinic to be connected to the HIE?

- ✔ How will lab results be received and interfaced — directly with labs (LabCorp, Quest, local labs) or via a local/regional/state HIE?

- ✔ How will the EHR send information to the state's immunization registry — via an interface or via HIE?

- ✔ How will the EHR send syndromic surveillance data to public health agencies — via an interface or via HIE?

- ✔ How will clinical summary information (problem list, medication list, allergies, and diagnostic test results) be exchanged among providers of care and patient authorized entities electronically using the CCD or CCR standard?

- ✔ What level of HIE integration is available within the EHR? Can HIE information be viewed within the EHR? Will patient and user context be shared or will a separate login be required?

- ✔ How will ambulatory quality measures be reported to CMS or the state to qualify for Medicaid or Medicare incentives?

Additionally, talk with outside lab companies to see whether they will cover interfaces to their organizations. Many do, but they may want to guarantee a certain number of transactions every month to make it worth their while. Ask whether the vendor has already implemented an interface with Quest, LabCorp, or your local HIE — if so, you're going to want to seek reduced costs (or no costs) for building the interface, as it has already been built.

Narrowing Your Vendor Choices

You don't have time to contact 400+ companies and review their systems, and even if you did, they all aren't a fit for you and your practice. So before you refine your list of potential partners, document what you need from a vendor partner. Focus on three topic areas as you develop your specific requirements:

- ✔ Functionality and workflow
- ✔ Information sharing
- ✔ Training and support

Use a formal request for information (RFI) to describe your needs and collect vendor information. After you know what you want and need, create a short list of vendors to contact and interview. Vendors are very accustomed to this process and should respond quickly to your request.

After receiving the vendor responses, cut the list one more time and decide which vendors you will invite to demonstrate their product. Ideally, limit the demos and site visits to three to five vendors. If you start to look at more than five, the products start to run together and you aren't making valuable use of your time.

Requirements gathering

Before you ask the vendors to support your needs, you have to know what you want and need. Fortunately, most specialties require the same general EHR functions to be successful. Table 6-2 lists the main capabilities and functionality that you'll most likely need from a vendor.

Table 6-2	Core EHR Functionalities
Functionality	*Notes/Details*
Documentation tools	Allow for multiple methods including free text, point and click, dictation, voice recognition, and use of macros
Clinical content	Templates, order sets, and letters
Order entry	Creating orders for labs, radiology studies, referrals, medications, and so on; links to problem list
Problem list management	ICD9; SnoMed; links to orders
Medication management	Reconciliation, historical capture, e-prescribing, and prescription writer

Functionality	Notes/Details
Results review	Lab, pathology, radiology — ability to trend, graph, and print
Referral management	Creation of referrals and managing incoming referrals
Telephone	Documentation and routing of patient telephone calls
Formulary management	Notification if medication is nonformulary based on patient's insurance
Health maintenance	Alerts for specific chronic diseases or suggested testing based upon age, sex, and history
Reporting	Manage a population of patients with a specific condition or disease
Clinical decision support	Alerts for interactions with drugs, food, allergies, and for duplicate ordering.
e-faxing	Communicate with outside providers
Cosigning and reviewing orders and notes	For mid-level providers, residents, and students
History documentation	Past medical, family, and social history with links to decision support and documentation
Patient education	Is it editable by the provider and in what languages can it be printed
Patient portal	Secure messaging, lab communication, immunization reports, and scheduling
E/M coding	Notification for missing information or education about requirements
Charge capture	Supplies and procedures

In addition to the core features, your practice has specific functions or workflows that an EHR must support. For example, you may need to document findings on body drawings within the EHR or input pictures of dermatological conditions and attach them to a patient's chart with your comments. Only you know exactly what you need. A potential vendor may be capable of serving in many capacities, but reading minds is probably not one of them. Make your needs known from the start. A vendor may not be able to satisfy all your requirements, but you'll never know if you haven't asked and described your practices in detail.

A connection from your EHR to the outside world provides great value in terms of efficiency and overall patient care. You want your vendor to support you in the most effective manner. You will save time and money if a vendor has experience interfacing with other systems you use. You may not know all the information about your system requirements, but the more you share with your prospective vendors, the more likely they'll meet your needs. Not a list maker? Well, it's time to become one. So, get out your scratch paper and put some thought into the following:

- ✔ The information systems that you are using, including practice management, scanning, and transcription
- ✔ The hospitals that you work with and their EHR systems
- ✔ Ancillary systems that you use, including labs, radiology, and therapy offices
- ✔ Other healthcare entities that you work with, including ambulatory surgery centers
- ✔ Key referral physicians and their EHR systems

Developing your RFI

A request for information (RFI) is a cover letter and overall description of your project goals that you send to vendors. Think of the RFI as the initial way to communicate some core data about you and your practice to the vendors to learn about how their products can best support you. Set a deadline for your vendors to return the RFI; two to three weeks is usually sufficient.

For each vendor, ask the same questions and capture the same information so that you can compare apples to apples and be fair in the process.

Practice information

Take the opportunity to describe your practice to the vendor. The more it knows about you, the better it will serve your needs. Provide the following information about your practice:

- ✔ Practice specialty, including single specialty versus multispecialty clinic
- ✔ Practice size and location, including working in multiple sites or needs for remote access from home
- ✔ Total number of employees by role
- ✔ Use of fellows, residents, medical students, nursing students, nurse practitioners, and physician assistants
- ✔ Primary language(s) of your patients
- ✔ Onsite resources, such as lab, radiology, and pharmacy
- ✔ Existing practice management system and other potential interface needs
- ✔ Existing computer hardware
- ✔ Current Internet network information (DSL, cable modem, T1, or none)

Vendor company information

Picking a vendor is more than just finding some product that has all the bells and whistles that you want. Inquire about the company and product history while you consider the viability and the growth of the vendor.

An unfortunate side effect of the surge in EHR interest is that vendors are finding it difficult to staff all of their implementations and meet their clients' needs in a timely manner. Becoming acquainted with a company's background before you choose your final partner is crucial to your EHR success.

Here is some good information to gather on each vendor:

- Company history, including founding year, growth, and public versus private status
- Acquisition history
- Number of employees, especially for development and client support
- Average experience (in years) for employees, with your company and within the industry
- Financial history of the company, with statements from the last three years
- History of the product
- Number of major upgrades in the last two years, including typical impact on a practice
- Listing of existing clients with size of practice, specialty, year implemented, and which EHR version the clients are using

Vendor functionality

All of your short-list vendors will support core EHR functionality (with rare exceptions), but they may accomplish the same task in different ways. Ask whether a key feature (to you) is being used by customers, in an upcoming release, or planned for development.

Additionally, you should ask about the core functionality and any specific features that meet your practice or specialty needs.

Vendor support and staff training

How the vendor supports you in the process of learning about and ultimately using the EHR effectively is just as important, if not more important, than functionality. Training is a vital element of vendor support, so ask these specific questions to assess how the vendor will train you and your staff now and in the long run:

✔ What are the training options for the EHR? Include expected time commitments, requirements by job role, timing of training, and methods.

For example, for a clinic with two physicians, three nurses, two front office staff members, and one billing staffer, how would you train them for an upcoming EHR and PM go-live?

✔ Do you provide, encourage, or require training post go-live? If so, describe the timing, length of training, cost, method of training, and content.

✔ Do you have e-learning or computer-based training (CBT) materials available? If so, describe what areas they cover, module lengths, and costs associated with their use.

✔ How do you train staff who are hired after a clinic's go-live? For example, say I hire a new physician and two new nurses six months after EHR implementation. Who trains those new clinicians? Is there an additional cost if you provide the training?

When you're ready to turn on the EHR and go-live, the vendor will likely have resources there to support you and your staff. Vendor support strategies vary with how long support remains onsite, when it returns, what resources it uses, and how ongoing maintenance is provided. No matter how well a vendor performs on day one, it won't always be perfect. Additionally, the vendor product will change and improve. Ask the vendor how it will help you optimize your system and learn new functionalities when they roll out.

Ask each vendor these questions:

✔ How do you support a clinic that is going live with EHR and PM applications?

✔ What resources do you provide during go-live?

✔ Are there different support packages? Describe the cost of each.

✔ How long does your support remain onsite?

✔ How do you support a clinic after the initial go-live period? Do you provide onsite resources post go-live?

✔ Is there an additional cost associated with onsite support?

✔ Are the resources from your company or are they a third-party contractor?

✔ Do you provide phone support?

✔ Do you provide Web support? If so, please describe.

✔ Is there a dedicated remote resource for the clinic or is there a call center?

✔ How do you process issues called in by a clinic, including how calls are handled and documented, the average response time for issues, and whether the clinic or end user can see where the issue is in the resolution process? What tools do you use to support this process?

✔ How would you support the following scenarios? Include types of resources that would help the clinic, any cost associated with the support, and length of the resolution process.

- A physician wants to add choices to physical exam or history questions.

- A physician wants to add new documentation templates.

- A nurse or physician is unable to find a specific lab or radiology test.

- A nurse or physician wants to add a new test to the order catalog.

- An interface to Quest or LabCorp is not functioning as expected.

- An interface to the hospital is not functioning as expected.

Asking for additional information

To complete the RFI, be sure to ask about the following:

✔ Any important topics or pertinent details unique to you or your needs. For example, in terms of benefits and return on investment data, you should ask for specific case studies if possible.

✔ Request a sample contract and the average length of time to complete contract negotiations.

✔ Any hardware and network requirements, remembering that the requirements are going to be different depending on whether you host the system.

✔ An implementation plan including average time from contract to go-live.

Creating a short list

You don't want to distribute your RFI to 400 vendors, so you should create a short list of vendors likely to meet most of your needs. Vendors target specific markets based on practice size and specialty. Use this information to help narrow the field. Combine your requirements with some industry information and identify no more than five vendors of the same type for the RFI distribution. Include the following vendors on your list:

✔ Vendors suggested by your colleagues.

✔ Vendors your hospitals recommend.

✔ Vendors recommended by your specialty society.

✔ Vendors your local HIE or Regional Extension Center supports. (If you're not sure how to contact the HIE, ask your local hospital's IT department or your Regional Extension Center.)

Review industry rating information from such groups as KLAS (www. klasresearch.com), peer-reviewed ratings at AmericanEHR Partners (www.americanehr.com), shown in Figure 6-1, or your specialty society. There is a fee for the full report from KLAS, but you can review the summary information on its Web site. You can find the latest year's ratings of ambulatory EHRs by practice size, too.

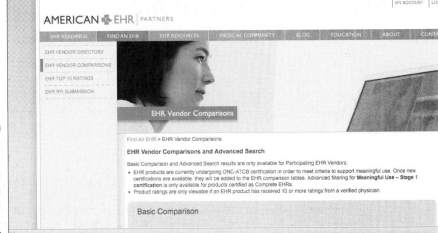

Figure 6-1: American-EHR Partners comparison engine.

Ideally, there should be a fair amount of overlap from all the sources so your list isn't unwieldy. Make a final list of three to five vendors and send your RFI with a cover letter to each one.

Deciding which products to see

Along with sending back the RFIs, vendors will likely send collateral material including books, CDs, and other marketing materials. Conduct both qualitative and quantitative analyses of the RFI information.

Create a master electronic file to store the RFI information so you can compare each vendor side by side that you feel is most important to you.

For the quantitative analyses, document the vendors' responses for each general category. For example, if there were 350 specific functionality questions and the vendor "meets requirements" or "functionality is live with clients" for 250 functionality points, document 71 percent.

Review the narrative responses, cost proposals, and collateral material as part of your qualitative analysis.

Set a meeting with the vendor selection team and present the case for each vendor. Using your agreed-upon decision process and all the information at your disposal, select no more than five vendors to continue in the selection process. Product demonstrations and site visits may be more time-consuming for your team, so limiting the number of vendors keeps the process manageable.

Getting the Pricing Right

Cost is a major part of your final decision, and understanding the total cost of ownership of the EHRs you're considering is important.

Comparing "apples and oranges"

Your RFI and evaluation process helps you compare needed functionality, but you need to make sense of the pricing. Often, vendor pricing is structured in a way that requires a decoder. Moreover, each vendor prices and packages its system differently. Understand what is and is not included in the vendor quote.

Here are a few line item costs to normalize across your quotes. Know whether these expenses are bundled with other costs or whether you'll be charged separately, and ensure you're looking at the same thing from each vendor:

- ✔ **Licensing**
  - Per provider upfront licensing fee (one time), if applicable
  - Per provider ongoing licensing fee (monthly, yearly)
  - Per provider licensing fee for practice management system, if applicable
  - E-prescribing licenses
  - Discounts, if applicable
  - Upgrades
- ✔ **Implementation and training**
  - Setup
  - Additional setup or customization
  - Onsite visits
  - Practice workflow redesign
  - Project management
  - Training

- Additional or customized training
- Go-live support
- Post go-live training

✔ **Data integration and interfaces**

- E-prescribing interface (to send and renew prescriptions electronically)
- Electronic eligibility checking
- Electronic claim submittal
- Automated remittance posting
- Practice management interface
- Document scanning interface
- Data migration of patients in your existing EHR or practice management system, if applicable
- Transcription and report interfaces (radiology reports)
- Electronic lab results interface (national labs, such as LabCorp and Quest; hospital labs; and local labs)
- Exchange of clinical summary information (using the CCD or CCR standard) for problem list, medication list, allergies, and diagnostic test results) among providers of care and patient-authorized entities
- Interfaces to local, regional, and state HIE

✔ **Ongoing operations and maintenance**

- Phone-based support during business hours
- Phone-based support outside normal business hours
- Monthly or annual maintenance fees
- Items that aren't covered by the maintenance contract
- Training new staff or physicians
- Retraining or additional training associated with upgrades or new releases
- Changes to interfaces (lab, radiology, transcription) due to upgrades and evolving Meaningful Use criteria

✔ **Add-ons and other applications**

- Patient portal, including patient-provider secure messaging
- Mobile application
- Telephone reminder system
- Patient education content or handouts

- Document management/scanning system
- Offsite backup, disaster/recovery services
- Migration to ICD10
- Anything else you see on a vendor's quote that you're not sure is included on another vendor's quote

Many costs of an EHR aren't included in the vendor's quote, such as hardware and getting your exam rooms ready for the computer. We discuss these considerations in Chapter 5. Make sure you have a sense of the total cost before going into contract negotiations with your vendor.

Comparing apples with apples

After you compare vendors, ask them to submit a Best and Final Offer to let your vendors know that you're serious about them, have done your homework, and have navigated through the marketing mumbo jumbo to figure out what's really being offered.

When asking for a Best and Final Offer, provide the vendors with a framework to follow. Tell vendors how you want them to list their pricing so that costs are broken down in a similar format for a normalized view that compares apples to apples.

Many Regional Extension Centers (RECs) have gone through this process and negotiated preferred pricing and contract terms. REC staff are also knowledgeable about what you may need and the services and solutions offered by EHR vendors. If your practice isn't served by a REC (you're not considered a priority primary care provider), many RECs still offer this information or assistance (free or at competitive costs) to practices interested in adopting EHRs. See Chapter 3 for resources that can help you through this.

Evaluating the System Demonstrations

When you trim your list of potential partners to three to five, you get to the fun part. You get to see (and, ideally, get your hands on) each system. Demonstration events should be informative and entertaining. Additionally, vendors may bring a lot of sizzle to their presentation; confirm which features are live and which have yet to roll out.

Take the opportunity to interview and interact with the vendor team during the demonstrations. This may be the only face-to-face interaction with potential vendors during the selection process. Therefore, use the experience to help influence your decision-making process.

Developing demonstration scenarios

Vendor demonstrations provide a great opportunity to see the products, meet the team, and "test drive" the system with your colleagues. Think of demos as EHR speed dating. All the vendors have their own scenarios and features that they want to show off. However, the demos are about how each product meets your specific practice needs.

Here are some simple guidelines for creating successful and useful demonstration scenarios:

- ✔ **Ask the vendor to demonstrate the functionality that is available and in use by other ambulatory practices.**

- ✔ **Request that each vendor be prepared to discuss his or her RFI responses.** Especially concerning (but not limited to) implementation timelines, support, training, pricing, interfaces, and overall integration.

- ✔ **Craft three to four reasonable clinical scenarios.** If you're part of a multi-specialty clinic, make sure to include scenarios from each specialty.

  Make sure that one or two of the scenarios are simple, straightforward patients. You want to see the efficiency of the system in action.

- ✔ **Create one or two clinically complex patient scenarios.** You want to see how the system can help you manage your real world patient in the 15-minute time slot you have.

- ✔ **Think about some of your difficult workflows, communications with patients, or general clinical quality.** Ideally, the EHR that you are choosing can help you solve some of your current woes.

- ✔ **Keep the scenarios consistent in every vendor demonstration.** You want to compare apples to apples.

- ✔ **Ask about every major functionality component that was on your list.** This is the best chance to see what the vendor described in its RFI response.

- ✔ **Spend time on everyone's role and not just the physicians.** Your entire staff has to work in the system, and if the front desk and nurses don't like the system, the physicians won't be happy either.

- ✔ **Keep your questions until the end of the demo.** Don't interrupt the vendors every few minutes. Allow them to get through an entire scenario or at least a major part of it without questions. Assessing the efficiency and flow of the system is very difficult if the vendor has to stop constantly.

- ✔ **Ask about planning, training, and support while you have the vendor team in front of you.**

- ✔ **Make sure the vendor has the functionality to back up a great-looking user interface.** Don't get mesmerized by the slickest and prettiest system.

Involving your staff and colleagues in the demos

The demonstrations offer the best and most tangible way to involve your colleagues and staff in the EHR selection process. Everyone wants to see the product they'll potentially be using every day, and reading through an RFI or looking at brochures just isn't the same as looking at the real thing.

Encourage at least one representative from each role to participate to ensure that you and the vendor focus on the entire patient and clinic experience. Having a physician thinking through the needs that a front desk staff member might have can be very difficult. Allow staff members to speak for themselves. Engaging the entire office in the process helps with picking the best EHR for the practice and helps with its adoption and use, too. To that end, you should have an audience at each demonstration to ensure equal comparisons and involvement. Arranging calendars might be difficult, so schedule the demos in advance and block time on everyone's schedule.

Scoring the demonstrations

Allow everyone who attends the demos to participate in the scoring. You may weigh the scoring differently for certain participants, but everyone should provide feedback. Use a standard form for each person and for each vendor to ensure consistency of the process. Additionally, the collection of the data and the scoring should be straightforward and easy to understand. Keep the process simple for a clearer and more enthusiastic response from your fellow team members. Figure 6-2 shows an example scoring form.

Your professional society or Regional Extension Center should have sample vendor demonstration scenarios and forms to help you.

Conducting site visits

The vendor demonstrations allow you to see the best and brightest features of the EHR products, but sometimes a presentation can feel too much like a sales pitch. Talk to other customers in their clinics, if possible. Although each clinic has its own special needs, the site visits provide an invaluable source of real-world experience that the demonstrations can't duplicate.

You do not need to include all your colleagues and staff from the demonstrations in the site visits. Identify two or three members of your team to make the trip and then communicate your findings to the rest of the team.

If you can't visit other clinics, then conduct phone interviews with their representatives. Telephone conversations with other sites are better than no interaction at all.

FUNCTIONALITY - The vendor strongly supports the following functions:	Strongly Agree +2 points	Agree +1 point	Unsure 0 points	Disagree -1 point	Strongly Disagree -2 points
A **Clinical Documentation & Review**					
A.1. Patient Lookup and Search					
A.2. Review of Patient Summary Information					
A.3. Encounter Note					
A.4. Progress/Consult Note					
A.5. Results Review (e.g., labs, radiology)					
A.6. Order Entry					
A.7. Electronic Prescribing					
A.8. Clinical Decision Support Alerts					
A.9. Consult and Referral Requests/Letters					
A.10. Modifying/Customizing Templates					
A.11. Chart Organization & Ease of Charting					
A.12. Remote Access					
B **Practice Coordination & Management**					
B.1. Practice Messaging and Tasking					
B.2. Telephone Message Documentation					
B.3. E/M Coding					
B.4. Charge Capture					
C **Patient Management & Communications**					
C.1. Reporting - Disease & Wellness Guidelines					
C.2. Meaningful User Reporting/Dashboard					
C.3. Patient Education					
C.4. E-visits, Secure Email with Patients					
Total Score					
D **Overall Impressions**					
D.1. I liked the following features:					
D.2. I am concerned about the following:					
D.3. Continue to consider this EHR (Yes/No)?					

Figure 6-2:
EHR vendor demonstration scoring sheet.

Here's how to find other clinics to visit:

- ✔ **Vendor-approved references:** Each vendor has a list of references and clinics willing to host site visits. Most will provide strong references; otherwise, they probably wouldn't be on the vendor's list. We're not suggesting that the sites would hide anything from you, but the vendor is going to provide sites where the implementations have gone well.

- ✔ **Doing your own reconnaissance:** Exploring local clinics is another option for site visits or visits to your colleagues' offices to hear their stories.

If a site isn't on the vendor's list of preferred references, the implementation could still be a success, but the clinic may not want to open its doors to outside groups.

If an implementation wasn't as successful as a site wanted, don't get discouraged. Inquire into why it didn't go well and what they would do differently.

Whether you're on the phone or conducting the site visit in person, be prepared to ask each site the same general questions about clinic and implementation history, the EHR itself, training and support, hardware and technology, and overall satisfaction. Here's a list of potential questions for each site reference:

- ✔ **Clinic and implementation history**

  - How many physicians, NPs, PAs, RNs, LPNs and front office staff are in your clinic?

  - What specialties practice in the clinic?

  - When did you go-live with the application?

  - What functionality did you go-live with?

  - Did you implement the vendor's practice management system? If not, does your system interface with the EHR?

  - Are you connected to your local hospital?

- ✔ **EHR**

  - Does everyone use the EHR? If not, why not?

  - Do you use voice recognition or dictation?

  - Can providers customize the system to meet their needs?

  - How long did it take to return to full productivity?

  - How much did you reduce your schedule at go-live?

  - Do you have access from the hospital or from home?

  - Have you identified any quality or patient care benefits as a result of the implementation?

  - Do your patients have access to the system?

  - How has EHR changed the role of the physician?

✔ **Training and support**

- Did you receive remote, onsite, classroom, or e-learning training?

- How many hours of training were needed for each role (physician, nurse, front desk)?

- Who provided the training?

- Did the vendor provide support at go-live? If so, for how many people and for how long? How effective was the vendor's go-live support?

- Did the vendor return after go-live for any additional training or support? If so, when and for how long?

- Does the vendor provide you remote support? If so, does it provide all the help you need?

- Do you and your colleagues feel like they are using the system to its fullest?

✔ **Hardware and technology**

- What type of devices do you use?

- If you had to pick devices again, would you use the same ones or pick something different?

- What recommendations do you have about device placement?

- Do you have any issues with connectivity or system responsiveness?

- Do you scan any information into the chart?

- Do you have any issues with interfaces to other systems in your clinic or outside the clinic?

- Does the vendor provide adequate support for your interfaces?

✔ **Overall satisfaction**

- Would you work with the vendor again?

- What would you do differently if you had to implement EHR again?

- Are you happy that you implemented EHR?

Making the Final Choice

Well, this may not necessarily be the absolute, final choice, but at this point, you should at least decide which vendor is your top choice. While you progress into the financial and contractual discussions, keep your second and third choices involved. Contract negotiations are challenging; having a backup option as leverage with your top choice (or if the whole deal falls apart) is valuable.

Document everything vendors do during the system demonstrations so you remember later. Their actions and words are a good indication of the partner they will be. Are they timely, respectful, and knowledgeable; or do you feel as if they're trying to sell you on the bigger and better deal?

Although system functionality is extremely important, how you and the vendor work together throughout your relationship has more to do with your success than a few well-placed system buttons. A vendor who goes out of its way for its clients' success can make up for a system that doesn't have every bell and whistle.

Weighting and scoring

Only you know how important each selection category is for your clinic. The EHR's functionality, the vendor's support, or the system and implementation costs might drive your decision. Each piece is critical to your success, but they don't measure equally. In consultation with the vendor selection team, determine a weight for each component and measure each vendor accordingly.

When you rate each product, consider your experiences with the vendors during the selection process. Use RFIs, collateral materials, demonstrations, site visit information, interviews, and industry experience to guide your choice. Also, factor how the vendor dealt with you and your staff, its responsiveness, its willingness to go the extra mile, and its knowledge of the EHR product and implementation. Figure 6-3 shows a sample vendor evaluation tool.

You can also calculate your overall score and determine your final vendor ratings by following these steps:

1. **Determine the weight for each selection category.**

2. **Collect and tabulate scoring sheets from each member of the selection committee.**

3. **Based on the weight each team member carries, calculate the final vendor score.**

Picking "the one"

After you tabulate the scores and determine the best fit for your practice, communicate your decision to each vendor. At this time, all but your top choice may offer you a better deal, negotiate special discounts, and bargain for another opportunity to get your business.

Evaluation Area (Rating Scale: 1 = Best, 4 = Worst)	Weight (%)	Vendor A Rank	Vendor B Rank	Vendor C Rank	Vendor D Rank
Clinical Functionality	20%	1	2	4	3
Ease & Speed of Review/Documentation	10%	2	1	3	4
Practice Management Integration	10%	4	1	3	2
Implementation & Training Approach	10%	1	2	3	4
Available Templates and/or Customization	10%	3	1	2	4
Ongoing Support - Online, Phone, On-Site	15%	1	2	4	3
Demonstration Rankings	10%	1	2	3	4
Reference Check/Site Visit Rankings	15%	2	1	4	3
Total	100%				

Evaluation Points Conversion: Rank 1 = 10 points   Rank 2 = 7 points
                                Rank 3 = 3 points   Rank 4 = 1 point

Vendor Rating Value: Weight X Evaluation Points

Evaluation Area	Weight	Vendor A Rating	Vendor B Rating	Vendor C Rating	Vendor D Rating
Clinical Functionality	20%	2	1.4	.2	.6
Ease & Speed of Review/Documentation	10%	.7	1	.3	.1
Practice Management Integration	10%	.1	1	.3	.7
Implementation & Training Approach	10%	1	.7	.3	.1
Available Templates and/or Customization	10%	.3	1	.7	.1
Ongoing Support - Online, Phone, On-Site	15%	1.5	1.05	.15	.45
Demonstration Rankings	10%	1	.7	.3	.1
Reference Check/Site Visit Rankings	15%	1.05	1.5	.15	.45
Total	100%	7.65	8.35	2.4	2.6

Figure 6-3:
An EHR vendor evaluation tool.

Allowing your top choices to one-up each other with better offers is tempting; however, trust your processes and the hard work you and your team just completed, and stick with your decision.

Nonetheless, document any new offerings or price breaks the runners-up offer because this information might be valuable during contract negotiations with your number one choice.

If you feel that there's still a good amount of negotiation that needs to happen before you sign on the dotted line with your preferred vendor — whether it's due to services or cost — then don't show all of your cards until it's the right time. It adds additional burden and coordination to your EHR selection process, so do this *only* if you feel that it's essential to get the terms you're seeking.

Inform Vendor A that it's your vendor of choice and that you're moving forward with contract negotiations, but still have a few items to iron out before you're ready to commit fully. Inform Vendor B that you've selected another vendor as your preferred vendor and are moving forward with contract negotiations, but that it is in second place and you may come back to them. Keep focused on Vendor A and proceed with contract negotiations, which you can read about in Chapter 7.

Chapter 7

Partnerships and Contracts

*Y*ou've played the field and flirted with the idea of working with different EHR vendors. You've dined with countless reps (on their dime, we hope), and participated in small talk on every topic from sports to the weather. And guess what — you're over it. Playing the EHR field is a lot of work, and you're ready to settle down.

When you've identified a vendor who you want to partner with, you're ready to start negotiating. Remember to keep your second and third choice informed of your progress in case you need some extra leverage during your negotiations with your first choice.

It's time to start living the rest of your clinical life in a paperless world, so get ready to hammer out the details of the contract that will govern your relationship. Let the negotiations begin!

Establishing a Sustainable Vendor Relationship

During the initial vendor selection phase, you started some serious conversations about what you and your clinic must have. You made your initial selection based on the vendor's ability to meet your needs and now you're ready to dive into next level of detail during this negotiation period. The more you know about the particulars of your vendor's technology requirements, implementation and migration services, industry reputation, and financial parameters, the smoother your negotiations and eventual long-term relationship. Continue to leverage outside resources like your local hospital and REC to help you get the best deal and navigate key discussion points. At the end of the day, you want the best deal possible that allows both you and the vendor to be successful.

One of the most important things to discuss with your vendor as part of the contracting process is their Meaningful Use readiness. Make sure you find out its preparedness to meet Meaningful Use requirements. Ask to see its official certification and any guarantees that it has to meet initial and ongoing MU requirements. Any incentive money you get back from the government depends on your EHR vendor meeting all necessary guidelines.

Make these conversations an important part of your presigning plans. It doesn't matter how difficult or challenging the conversation may be; what matters is that you have it. Do whatever you have to do — buy lunch or set up teleconferences — to cover vital information and deal breakers with your vendor rep.

Technology requirements

The first item to discuss with your vendor is your technology needs. You want to make sure that everything you think is true about your practice's technological plusses and minuses is, in fact, true. Confirm hardware and software with your vendor rep to assure everyone's on the same page. Here are some initial questions to cover with your rep:

- ✔ What hardware do we need to replace or upgrade? And does the vendor offer any special hardware pricing as part of its contract?
- ✔ Do we need a different contract with an Internet service provider or network?
- ✔ In addition to adding the EHR, will we need to change, add, or upgrade other software programs?
- ✔ What interfaces are recommended by the vendor and what experience does it have with your other systems (practice management, Lab Corp, Quest)?
- ✔ Who pays for the interfaces and who does the work on the interface development?
- ✔ What kind of software licenses do you offer?
- ✔ What happens if the EHR system experiences a failure?
- ✔ How does your disaster recovery system work?
- ✔ How often can we expect software upgrades and will we have to pay for them?
- ✔ Do you currently or have plans to integrate with a personal health record (PHR) into the existing EHR? If so, what is your timeframe and how will that affect our practice?
- ✔ Are there any functionalities or features of the software that are considered extras?

Migration and implementation services

Now is also the time to ask any final questions and set expectations about how best to handle migration of data from paper records to the EHR system and confirm what implementation services will be included in your contract. Ask your rep:

- ✔ What kind of support will you offer while we preload data from paper records into the EHR?

- ✔ Do you offer data conversion services if we don't want to do the preloading?

- ✔ How long will preloading of key patient information take?

- ✔ Will you or our practice take the lead for the implementation?

- ✔ How much time will we need to devote to implementation?

- ✔ Do you offer alternative implementation schedules so we don't disrupt patient flow?

- ✔ Can you run parallel systems during the go-live phase in case we experience glitches with the new EHR?

- ✔ What kind of implementation and training materials do you provide?

Financial parameters

You already know what sorts of costs you will incur with EHR adoption and implementation. However, you're bound to run into a fair amount of fine print when it comes time to signing the contract. To avoid any big, earth-shaking surprises, make sure you understand the financial expectations of migrating to EHR. Discuss the following with your vendor rep prior to making your relationship official:

- ✔ How do software license fees work? Do we have to purchase multiple licenses or renew them at any time? Are the licenses sold per practice, physician, or user? How do you account for part-time employee usage?

- ✔ How do you provide access to databases, such as code sets or journals? Is there a license that we must pay for, or is access included in your overall cost?

- ✔ What is covered under your standard maintenance policy? Is there anything we have to pay extra for to have serviced?

✔ What support is included in your package?

✔ Will there be regular updates or enhancements that we have to purchase, or are they optional?

✔ How much does having you preload existing charts cost?

✔ What is your best estimate of the cost for loss in productivity during implementation and go-live? Get the vendor's estimate, based upon actual experience, on how long your reduced patient load will last.

Legal stuff

Always ask the vendor rep about your legal rights. You (or one of your teammates) have made sure that you're hooking up with a reputable vendor that will do right by you if things go south. This conversation, however, should focus on your legal rights in terms of data storage and usage and what happens if your system experiences a catastrophic failure. Ask your vendor:

✔ Are there provisions in the contract about proprietary information? What are they?

✔ For claims and personal health information, how is "ownership" defined?

✔ Who determines the parameters of data access and termination procedures?

✔ What are your procedures for data recovery?

✔ What is the coverage for system failure because of software glitches; user error; or an unforeseen event, such as a fire or an electrical failure?

✔ What do your liability provisions cover? What do you expect our insurance to cover? Will you agree to cover loss above and beyond the software?

✔ What happens if you go out of business? Can you agree to provide us with any legal recourse if patient data needs to be migrated to another system or re-entered by our team?

✔ What kind of indemnity can you offer to cover our practice if a software-based coding malfunction causes Medicare or Medicaid to investigate us?

✔ How do you handle a breach of confidentiality?

✔ Does your insurance company have a liability cap for third parties?

✔ How do you structure your indemnification process to determine who has responsibility for any future legal action or fines?

✔ Is there a force majeure clause to limit any liability or obligation in the event of extraordinary events or circumstances outside of both group's control?

Discussing your security concerns

To have a successful, sustainable vendor relationship, you must talk with your rep about your security concerns. Patients are bound to have security questions when you transition to EHR; keep security paramount for their well-being and the longevity of your practice.

This is the time to be candid — no question is out of bounds, especially if the vendor wants to ensure your level of comfort with the provided security measures. Though much of the onus to protect patient information is on the vendor and its software, the responsibility for maintaining data integrity is ultimately yours. Be sure your rep is knowledgeable about the software's security features and how they'll protect you during a security breach.

Knowing what kind of security coverage a vendor provides across office lines is vital. Because many stakeholders access your practice's EHR data to provide patient care, all kinds of employees have contact with your patients' health data. Ask your vendor to sign a *Business Associate Agreement,* which ensures that your practice and EHR support HIPAA (Health Insurance Portability and Accountability Act). Your practice is held accountable for following HIPAA privacy guidelines, and you have to feel comfortable with your vendor's level of compliance. Find out whether the vendor is up to speed on all of the latest HIPAA rules and regulations and that its software reflects a commitment to privacy and security. A Business Associate Agreement ensures that all parties with access to patient health information agree to protect this private information and use it only for intended and specified purposes.

Your vendor should be willing to participate in an audit for compliance with HIPAA privacy and security rules.

Other security issues that you should address with your vendor prior to signing any paperwork include

- ✔ **Termination and security:** If a vendor goes out of business, will it be willing to work with you during the phase-out period to show you how to retrieve and save EHR information?

- ✔ **Preloading and shredding security:** Will the vendor assist you with understanding the proper handling of paper records during the preloading phase and the disposal phase?

- ✔ **Encryption:** Have the vendor rep explain the software encryption coding to you. Even if you feel like this is too techy, take thorough notes so you can relay the information to your staff and any outside IT professionals.

EHR contract negotiations can take roughly 2–3 months, so be ready to hunker down.

If your EHR isn't in compliance with HIPAA, then your practice isn't compliant with HIPAA. Being out of compliance with HIPAA can involve penalties, both civil and criminal, punishable by fines or imprisonment. Civil financial penalties can range from $100 to $25,000 per year for the same violation. Fines for a criminal offense for disclosing or misusing personal health information are substantial, ranging from $50,000 to $250,000 and one to ten years in prison. Be absolutely certain, before you sign any contracts, that your vendor can keep you HIPAA-compliant.

Asking about support and update practices

Your vendor relationship does not end after go-live. You and the vendor are in this thing for the long haul, so you should account for the fact that people and situations change. What works for your EHR software today may be obsolete in five years. So spend some time finding out about the support and update options your vendor provides. You spend a great deal of time researching, training, preloading, and implementing — you also want to keep your software humming along and as current as possible.

If your vendor rep is unsure about the ongoing support services the vendor provides or cannot provide you with details about how updates and upgrades are implemented, you may want to rethink your choice. Support and update practices are vital to the longevity and health of your EHR, so you have to find a vendor who takes system maintenance as seriously as you do.

When you sit down for your EHR heart-to-heart, confirm the following with your vendor rep:

- How often is the system upgraded and is there a regular release schedule?
- Are there any costs associated with an upgrade?
- Will the vendor supply any support resources for training with any major upgrade?
- What steps will the vendor take to ensure regulatory compliance?
- Will the vendor provide regular software upgrades or updates based on legislation?
- Does the vendor have a typical Service Level Agreement detailing customer service hours and procedures for system and technical issue resolution?
- What level of hardware maintenance is provided?
- What are the standard maintenance fees and what's included in those fees?

Agreeing to Terms and Getting Them in Writing

You may find this surprising, but many EHR vendors aren't used to vigorous contract negotiations with potential clients, particularly physicians. They do, however, have a lot of experience in negotiating with larger hospital systems and other large-scale providers. But as for you and your relatively small practice, negotiating much beyond the parameters of the boilerplate contract is rare. That's certainly not to say that you shouldn't make the effort to negotiate any points you wish — you should; and be firm about what it is you want from the EHR provider.

Consider the vendor rep your ally in negotiating final terms. After all, he or she wants to get a sale and form a long-lasting business relationship as much as you want to lose paper records and migrate to an EHR.

Everyone wins, as long you can hammer out the following details:

- ✔ **License fees:** These fees depend on how many providers you have in the office, according to the vendor's definition of provider. For example, your number of providers could be based on how many physicians you have in the office. Or it may be based on the combined number of doctors, nurse practitioners, and assistants. There are three types of pricing:

    - *Tiered pricing:* Doctors pay a higher price than nurses or front/back office staff

    - *Site license:* If your practice has more than 25 providers

    - *Enterprise license:* If you have multiple users in multiple environments

- ✔ **Meaningful Use:** Your federal incentive dollars are directly tied to your EHR certification and Meaningful Use of the system. Have the vendor confirm in writing that the software is in compliance with all certification benchmarks and Meaningful Use criteria *in perpetuity* (forever). Make sure, too, that the vendor offers compensation in the event it fails to meet requirements that are, at the very least, related to your lost incentive payments or penalties you incur.

- ✔ **Support terms:** Though support can be defined in all sorts of ways, how the vendor helps you keep the EHR running optimally (and what they will do for you if it fails) is what's important. Be specific here; ask that your vendor include even the smallest support detail in writing, including what penalty they will pay if they fail to provide those supports.

✔ **Updates:** Agree on what constitutes an upgrade as well as how and when you will be notified of available updates and upgrades to the EHR software. The last thing you want is to purchase an EHR, go through the implementation and go-live phases and, a few months later, find that the vendor requires you to upgrade the software. Get a firm answer about the vendor's upgrade plans to make sure you won't get burned in the short term. If the vendor is planning to require an upgrade within the year, consider waiting before you sign.

✔ **Provisions for vendor failure or consolidation:** What happens to your data if the vendor shutters operations or is bought by another vendor? Include a line item that details the contingency plan the vendor will provide so that your data remains secure and accessible during the transition and after you sign with a new vendor. Be sure the vendor can answer whether you will have to re-license software in the event of a consolidation and how to handle a new vendor that doesn't support your practice's platform.

✔ **Payment structure:** This is when you find out just how agreeable your vendor really is. Ideally, you want to set up the payment terms that best fit your financial scenarios. However, the vendor wants to get paid as soon as possible. Plan on agreeing to pay a portion of the total cost up front, another payment after installation, and a final payment after go-live.

Introducing the Service Level Agreement (SLA)

Think of a Service Level Agreement (SLA) as a prenuptial for the services provided to your clinic. You would use an SLA if you want to spell out the levels, limits, and quality of the vendor's promised services. Additionally, an SLA should consolidate the various vendor services into performance levels (standard or optional), assign resource commitments to your level of expectation, and name the services offered by the vendor in your overall contract.

The SLA can have several different points of negotiation, depending on your clinical situation. Some potential items up for negotiation include

✔ **Technology**

- Hardware or software
- Response times
- Bandwidth
- Throughput
- Configuration standards

- Downtime/uptime
- Documentation
- Planning assistance

✓ **Support**
- Methods
- Services
- Availability
- Response times
- Approved security levels

✓ **Maintenance**
- Upgrades and updates
- Patches and performance stability
- Software releases

✓ **Training**
- Training materials
- Onsite instruction
- Offsite instruction

✓ **Data**
- Integrity
- Conversion or migration
- Loss and recovery
- Protection

An SLA can be as thorough as you want it to be. However, if you add some vendor services to your final contract that aren't detailed in the SLA, they're considered mere options. Like any other agreement, the SLA works as a fluid document that is open to modification as technologies evolve.

Developing a Successful Contract

After you have all the difficult conversations and double- and triple-check all the contract terms, you put all of that hard work into motion and create the final contract.

Your vendor will most likely offer a boilerplate contract that includes terms favorable to — big surprise — the vendor. Don't be shocked or offended by this; the vendor is doing exactly what you're doing — looking out for its own business interests. Negotiation is expected, so be ready to dig in and push the vendor to include terms that favor your practice. Get a lawyer involved to review and edit your contract; you'll find that it's a great investment in the long run. The following sections outline some steps to take when creating the EHR contract.

Reading the boilerplate

The first step is to read the basic contract the vendor gives you. This document will include *boilerplate,* or standard language and terms set forth by the vendor. You'll probably see the following information in most EHR vendor contracts:

- ✔ Definitions
- ✔ Fees — licensing, interfaces, maintenance
- ✔ Licensing terms
- ✔ Payment terms
- ✔ Service Level Agreement for maintenance and support
- ✔ System availability, uptime, and response time
- ✔ Upgrades and future release versions
- ✔ Training
- ✔ Business Associate Agreement for HIPAA compliance
- ✔ Data Use Agreement
- ✔ Data ownership
- ✔ Confidentiality
- ✔ Liability
- ✔ Breach remedies
- ✔ Dispute resolution
- ✔ Indemnification
- ✔ Termination
- ✔ Third-party software
- ✔ Legal and regulatory information
- ✔ Meaningful Use guarantee or warranty
- ✔ Warranty

Marking up the contract

This point in the process is where you get to use a red pen. Make copies for your transition team of the vendor's initial contract and start marking it up. Write questions in the margins, mark places where you need clarification, and cross out any terms that you absolutely do not want to include. No one else is going to see your messy, marked-up version of the contract, so give yourself permission to make as many notes as necessary. It is probably a good idea to shred it when you're done unless you feel the need to keep it for posterity. Here are some points that you absolutely want to make sure the contract includes:

- Bilateral termination clause with no penalty and a specified time period
- Nontransferable by one party without written approval of the other party
- Definitions for any terms that may not be easily understood
- Evenly weighted contract default terms
- Delivery details (local hosting or ASP)
- Responses to RFIs
- Data ownership and access terms
- Minimum hardware requirements
- Hardware and software upgrade details
- Provisions for vendor failure or termination
- Cost for additional upgrades
- Cost associated with third-party software
- Confidentiality assurance
- Assurance that vendor complies with state and federal requirements
- Procedures for changes and updates, including timelines
- Provisions for ability of data to be separated if multiple practices will use the same system
- Payment schedules
- Conditions that constitute a breach of contract by either party
- Support terms
- Interface specifications
- Training details and costs
- Implementation details and costs
- Disaster recovery and planning

This is not necessarily the end-all, be-all contract checklist, but — at the very least — you should make sure these elements are at addressed in the contract. If not, it's back to the negotiating table for you.

Negotiating and renegotiating

After you work your magic with that red pen, go back to the vendor rep and hammer out the final details of the contract. You and the vendor have talked through all the details and agreed to all the terms and conditions. If there were any miscommunications or misinterpretations about terms, this is your last chance to make your voice heard and get what you want from the vendor (at least from a contract standpoint). So make any final demands or requests at this point and get it in writing.

You can still walk away at this point. Until you sign on the dotted line, your business is up for grabs, even if you have gotten this far with a vendor. Nothing is final until *you* say it is.

Signing your life away

Ready the trumpets and pour the champagne. If all has gone to plan, you've negotiated contract terms that benefit your practice most and reached an amicable compromise on points that aren't 100 percent in your favor. You can finally trade in your red pen for that nice, fancy Cross or Mont Blanc pen and sign that contract!

Flying with the legal eagles

Hopefully, your practice has a lawyer on retainer to handle issues of malpractice and more general legal concerns. If so, great, because you will probably want a legal representative to review the contract to make sure you are covered in case liability or compliance issues pop up.

If you don't have permanent counsel on retainer or your attorney is not well-versed in healthcare IT issues, then contact your REC, your professional society, an EHR consultant, or a software procurement professional who speaks the healthcare IT language. Because IT-related contracts can be complicated, especially for people who don't normally deal in technology, you might miss some of the finer points of the terms you're negotiating. Having a lawyer is a great step toward getting the most favorable terms for your practice. And employing an attorney who specializes in technology negotiations so you can garner the best terms is a bonus. A lawyer adds to your final list of costs, but might pay for himself by getting you the best deals. You want terms that you can live with for the long term, so lawyer up if you have the funds. Contact your colleagues and local RECs for assistance in locating lawyers who specialize in technology contracts. See Chapter 3 for a list of RECs.

The EHR contract is considered legally binding as soon as all parties sign. So, again, we advise you, your transition team, and your legal representative to re-read the contract to make sure all your requirements are spelled out. When you confirm they are, sign that baby and take a big, cleansing breath. You just bought an EHR!

Structuring Payment Terms and Models

Your new partner in practice life, the EHR vendor, wants to be paid. And because it wants to keep your business, it will likely work with you to hammer out a payment structure that's beneficial for it and your cash flow. Although overall EHR price is important, the payment structure is even more vital to your practice's sustainability.

You have to pay some money up front. Most EHR vendors require some sort of down payment, ranging from $500 to $15,000, depending on your time frame, practice size, and technology needs. Even though the software as a service (SaaS) model is becoming more popular — where you're mostly paying monthly fees — there are often upfront costs for data migration, interface development, and system implementation. Beyond that, you can work with the vendor to create payment terms and timeframes that will help you pay for the EHR, along with all your other bills. Some possibilities to consider include

- ✔ One hundred percent payment upfront.
- ✔ Partial payment upfront, followed by milestone payments. These might be based on different implementation phases — payment at time of contract signing, completion of preloading data, completion of training, and post go-live.
- ✔ Payments tied to receipt of your incentive money.
- ✔ Payments associated with the vendor's responsibility for helping your practice reach Meaningful Use.
- ✔ Payments associated with Meaningful Use guarantees set forth in the contract.
- ✔ Monthly or quarterly maintenance fees.
- ✔ Payments for upgrades or license renewal made upfront or at time of service.
- ✔ Lump sum payment for tech support.
- ✔ Yearly tech support fee or bills sent following individual tech support visits.
- ✔ Support fees paid upon service delivery or at time of continued training sessions.

✔ Support fees based on response times.

✔ Penalties associated with failure to deliver support, technical service, or appropriate upgrades or updates.

Ownership of data is a big issue, so make sure that you understand who owns the data contained in your EHR — your practice or the vendor. Consider adding financial provisions so you're compensated for any misuse of data if the vendor goes under or is sold.

Pinching contractual pennies

When you negotiate your payment terms, that is also a great time to think about ways you can save costs on your EHR. You've probably prioritized the features you want from a vendor, but if any of those are cost-prohibitive, you might be able to brainstorm ways to cut costs in other areas. Try these tips to stretch an EHR buck:

✔ Join a purchasing group to get a discount.

✔ If you're a primary care provider, contact your local REC for preferred pricing. If you're not a primary care provider, ask your local REC whether you can take advantage of this pricing.

✔ Find out if non-doctors can get a reduced licensing fee.

✔ Work with your lab or other outside colleagues to find out how their interfaces work, and see whether they will cover any additional costs associated with interfacing different systems.

✔ Buy hardware from a bulk purchasing group.

✔ Negotiate favorable return timeframes, up to 60 or 120 days post-purchase.

✔ Include hardware training in your purchase agreement.

✔ Purchase a maintenance agreement for all software, including peripherals.

✔ Negotiate a multiyear contract with your Internet provider to reduce fees.

✔ Ask your Internet service provider to include additional support services.

✔ Negotiate for a monthly service contract instead of an hourly rate.

✔ Include additional training hours when you negotiate the license agreement so you don't get slammed with more expensive add-on training hours.

✔ Request access to online tutorials and webinars.

✔ Barter vendor implementation hours for more training.

✔ Ask for the next few major upgrades to be included in your initial purchase price.

✔ Share hardware and IT support with other practices in your referral network.

✔ Hire an intellectual property attorney to save you money down the road.

Part III

I've Bought a System, Now What? Implementing an EHR

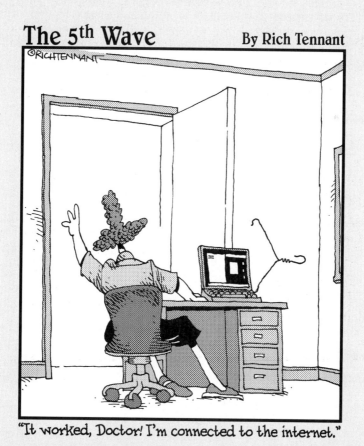

The 5th Wave   By Rich Tennant

"It worked, Doctor! I'm connected to the internet."

In this part . . .

Here you get to find out what all of this EHR hype really means to your organization. Chapter 8 helps you plan for your new workflow redesign. Chapter 9 is all about people — who will do what job and what new responsibilities and opportunities exist in an EHR environ- ment. Chapter 10 covers privacy and how to make your EHR secure while providing ample notification to your patients. Chapter 11 guides you through the major aspects of training and making training work for you. Chapter 12 opens the lines of communication, literally, and helps you find ways to inform staffers, colleagues, and patients about your new EHR. Chapter 13 is your go-to guide for surviving the always-exciting period known as go-live.

Chapter 8

Changing the Way You Work: Workflow Redesign

*E*HR is all about changing how your practice does business. Transitioning to the EHR is going to change your practice's day-to-day functions in several ways, from providing more patient information earlier in your clinical decision-making process to freeing up the space that used to be occupied by paper record storage. Your practice is going to run leaner and meaner. (Not *mean* meaner. You'll still be nice — we promise.) And, after everyone adjusts to the new way of office life that electronic records provide, you'll enjoy the benefits of your hard work during the research, transition, and go-live phases. One of the biggest benefits of converting to the EHR is streamlining your workflow so you can save time and provide a better quality of care for your patients.

Remember the core components that make up a workflow: people, process and technology. You impact all three areas while you redesign your practice.

Rethinking Your Workflow

There are almost as many reasons to redesign your workflow as there are steps you take to perform each daily task. When you rethink your practice's workflow design, you can identify opportunities for improvement that are possible with the EHR. You can also improve office practice efficiency, improve outcomes and the EHR design and adoption, reduce or eliminate non–value-added activities, identify and leverage parallel actions, and standardize procedure throughout the clinic.

A bad paper process won't improve just by adding technology; you only end up with a bad technical process. Spend the time to think about how you can change workflows beyond the computer screen.

There are all sorts of ways to improve workflow, and companies use a variety of workflow improvement theories to help them re-vision their processes and procedures. Some of the most popular include

- **Six Sigma:** Improves workflow quality by identifying and eliminating the causes of defects while minimizing variability. If you've ever heard someone say they are a "black belt," they are trained in Six Sigma.

- **LEAN:** Production practice that considers spending resources for any goal other than creating value for the end consumer wasteful and identifies targets for elimination.

- **LEAN Six Sigma:** If LEAN and Six Sigma had a baby, it would look like this: A combination of creating more value with less work and eliminating production process defects.

- **Total Quality Management (TQM):** Improves quality by ensuring compliance with internal requirements.

- **Business Process Reengineering:** The analysis and redesign of workflow between enterprises.

- **Plan-Do-Check-Act (PDCA):** This process improvement system focuses on solving business process improvement problems.

One or more of these processes may be best for your practice, or perhaps you wish to wing it and make up your own methodology for workflow redesign. Because you conducted the initial research necessary to begin your EHR journey, you should have quite a file of information about your workflows. Refer to some of the answers you accumulated during the readiness assessment, and you can apply your understanding of EHRs and your practice workflow to see how your workflows can change for the better.

You don't have to change the way you do everything in the office, but using your EHR does mean you have to make some changes. Make the changes work for you and your employees by addressing how you perform the work now, how you want to improve that workflow, and how EHR can help you make it happen.

All this workflows and processes talk is wonderful and useful. But none of it will matter if you don't have enough room to actually *do* the work. If you can evaluate your office layout now, you can avoid any nasty surprises about what will or won't fit on the day you reconfigure the space to make room for the EHR. Be sure to consider the following:

- ✔ **Power needs:** What will you need to plug in and where?

- ✔ **Office furniture:** How will you store or display hardware devices?

- ✔ **Storage room needs:** Where will you put extra devices, server, networking equipment? Is new space needed?

- ✔ **Ideal layout:** If you could reconfigure where desks, walls, and outlets are, how would you do it?

- ✔ **Room design:** How would you design the exam rooms to make space for new equipment?

- ✔ **Patient communication:** How will you ensure that you can communicate effectively with the patient while still using the EHR?

- ✔ **New uses for file room space:** What will you do with the space being used to house paper records?

You can create a quick diagram of your office layout using existing blueprints (like the one in Figure 8-1), or just eyeball it. This doesn't have to be to scale. Make several copies and use individual ones to draw in the various ways you'll use the space. You could, for example, draw where the current hardware resides or where you hope to place the new workstations. You can use the blueprint to track the life of a chart during a typical visit to see how you can improve workflow. You're only limited by your imagination here, so get some drawing pencils and spend some time playing Picasso. Who knows what you'll discover?

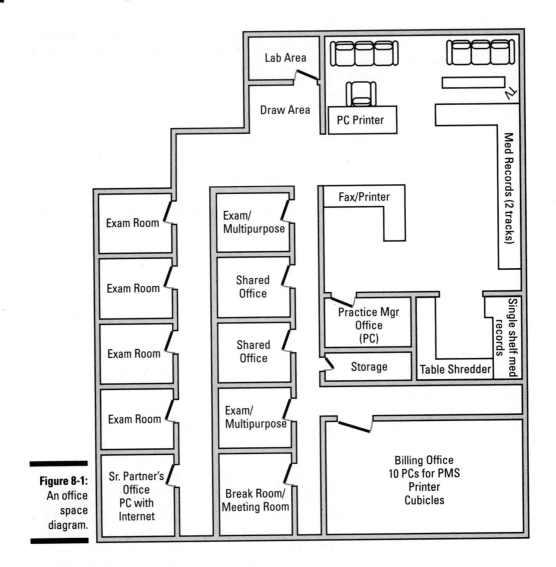

Figure 8-1:
An office space diagram.

Knowing How Your Practice Really Works

Step 1 of the workflow redesign process is to familiarize yourself with your workflows. We would say "refamiliarize" because you have to revisit procedures that may seem rote to you. Documenting and analyzing the tasks you do every day might seem like a lot of work, but, truth is, because you've been doing these workflows repeatedly, they've become second nature to you, easily forgettable, and difficult to change.

For example, say that you've brewed your own coffee for years, the same way every time. You probably don't even consider there could be a better way to make coffee. Then, one day, your spouse adds a half scoop more coffee and a pinch of cinnamon. Hello, flavor explosion! Suddenly, you see what you've been missing for years, simply because you never thought there could be a better way to make coffee.

Think about workflow design in the same way, and consider the possibility that maybe a process *can* be improved. When conducting an assessment of your workflows, you can be as formal or as informal as you like. If you choose to go the formal route, you can use the business process modeling notation (BPMN), or also more simply known as *process mapping*. These are just ways to describe flowcharts that represent the workflows in your practice. Figure 8-2 shows a flowchart.

You certainly don't have to be that formal in reviewing your workflows, although these more complicated methods might give you some workflow topics to address you hadn't thought of. To do a similar, but more informal, analysis, you can always set up a simple flowchart for each workflow. Or if designing flowcharts isn't your thing, you can always opt for the step-by-step method, in which you simply list the steps necessary to complete each task.

Track the time it takes to complete each step in a workflow and document baseline measurements as a part of your analysis. Knowing how long it takes to check in a patient or room a patient, for example, can help you find trouble spots in your processes. It will also help you after the go-live when you're trying to determine whether the EHR is making you more efficient or slowing you down. Having the analysis done beforehand will allow you to objectively review your post go-live activities.

Regardless of your analysis method, you need to look at how your practice works pre-EHR so that you can pinpoint areas to improve in your main work-flow categories. Whether you opt for the flowchart method or choose to write steps, you should ask some questions while you perform your analysis. When thinking about your questions, categorize your practice workflows in a way that works for you: by area of the office, by employee function, or by task. The following sections organize workflows into categories of patient flow, visit documentation, after visit communications, and document management.

Patient flow

How efficiently you move patients through the practice's office each day depends largely on how smoothly your workflow is designed. Now you don't necessarily want to move patients through your office like it's a drive-thru window. (Here's your lab result. Would you like fries with that?) But you do want to reduce wait times and create a smoother flow of people and proce-dures in the practice's office.

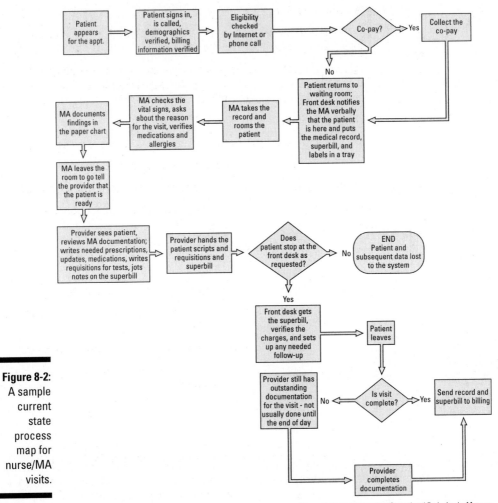

Figure 8-2: A sample current state process map for nurse/MA visits.

From a Systems Approach to Operational Redesign by Masspro

Recognize that your patients' time is as valuable as your own. Work to create a patient flow model that offers patients with the least time spent waiting and the most face time with physicians.

You may be surprised to find while you note the state of your patient flow affairs that you come up with a lot of "Why?" questions. For example, maybe you've always had the same employee conduct patient intake. Why is that? Perhaps you can think of a way to either share that responsibility or to assign it to another team member if that makes more sense. Ask yourself (and your team members) these questions to get a firm idea of how your patient flow is moving through your clinic:

✔ **Pre-visit and check in**

- What types of appointment require different blocks of time (e.g., new patient, physical, follow-up)?

- What information do we ask for, review, or provide before the patient visits the practice (appointment reminders, viewing patient information, diagnostic follow-ups)?

- How do we handle "no-shows"?

- What information does the patient provide at check-in?

- What documents (if any) are scanned at check-in?

- Does the patient make a co-payment at check-in or check-out?

- Does the patient sign a medical release or HIPAA form at check-in?

✔ **Rooming a patient**

- Who accompanies the patient while they move throughout the office?

- How does the clinical staff know a patient has arrived?

- If tests are performed before the provider meets with the patient, how are results communicated?

- How is the provider notified that a patient is ready to be seen?

- How is the provider notified of information captured by the nurse or medical assistant when rooming the patient, such as reason for visit, vitals, and medications or allergies reviewed?

✔ **Provider visit**

- Does the provider review patient information prior to or after entering exam room? If so, what information is typically reviewed?

- Where and how is the active patient medication and diagnoses lists documented and managed? (Is there summary information kept on the front of the chart or front cover?)

- How does the provider write orders for labs, radiology studies, referrals, and medications? (Orders may be different for each type of test.)

- Where and how are charges captured for each patient visit?

- What patient education materials are offered and by whom?

- Who performs minor in-office procedures, such as immunizations?

- How does the provider notify patients of a need for follow-up (appointment, test, referral)?

✔ **Check-out**

- What information does the patient bring to the front desk at check-out?

- How do you schedule future appointments (at check-out, postcard reminder, e-mail reminder)?

- Do you schedule appointments for other providers/specialists or for tests?

- Who faxes prescriptions to the pharmacy?

- How are charges handled after the patient leaves the office?

Though many of these questions may seem to have obvious answers, you may be surprised at some of your findings. Remember that any information you glean here is good information — don't make any assumptions about your workflows until you review your answers. Concentrate on documenting what the task is; who performs the task; what, if any, tools the task requires, and whether the task's process could be improved. Remember that improved workflow has three components: people, process, and technology.

Visit documentation

Not surprisingly, there's quite a lot of paperwork associated with each patient visit. The majority of this documentation occurs where the physician (or other medical personnel) provides care because the (often, one) paper chart is usually with the patient. What once was documented on paper is now documented using your EHR software. Aside from spending less money on paper products, you and your staff will have to maximize your functional mobility and make the most accurate notes for each patient visit. But first, think about how you perform documentation.

Providing documentation using the EHR isn't just about using less paper, it's also about providing a better quality of care for patients and a better quality of life for providers and office staff.

Ask yourself and your team some initial questions to define documentation patterns and preferences. Doing so can help you determine how you can best use the EHR and associated hardware devices (such as workstations) and mobile computing devices (such as laptops or tablets). Here are some questions to get you started:

✔ What portions of each patient visit are documented?

✔ Who documents patient information?

✔ What is documented while a patient is being placed in an exam room?

- Recording vitals

- Medication and history review

- Protocol orders and results (for example, a urinalysis for an OB patient)

✔ What is documented by the nurse or medical assistant and by the physician after the patient is in the exam room?

- Where does the nurse or medical assistant documentation occur?

- Where does the physician documentation occur (the exam room with the patient, the physician's office, or in a hallway)?

- When is the patient documentation completed?

- How is documentation completed (handwritten notes or transcription?

✔ Is any documentation completed after the patient visit? If so, how, where, and by whom?

Just popping in: Even quick visits have workflows

Reviewing your processes for patient flow during the standard office visit makes sense. But, what about those times when a patient drops by for a quick test or needs to drop off his latest glucose numbers for the physician to review? You still need to review the workflow design for the smallest of visits.

For example, if a patient is coming in for a blood pressure check with a nurse, you can note whether the check-in or rooming process differs from a physician visit and what the differences are. List the possible reasons — immunization, patient education, ear irrigation, and so on — that a patient might visit with a nurse or other staff member (lab technician, nurse educator) instead of a physician and whether the documentation differs. List any ways that protocols and forms for ordering tests by a nurse and a practitioner differ. Do the charge captures differ? Basically, find out whether non-physician visits differ from physician visits and, if so, how.

You could also run a workflow check on how, say, you handle times when patients pop in unannounced or even when (and this is rare) patients come in with a condition that requires emergency medical attention. Addressing your alternate patient visit scenarios will give you a fuller picture of how your staff can roll with the changes.

While you capture information related to your documentation habits, think of opportunities to improve and streamline each process. Here are some additional questions to ask yourself and your staff:

- ✔ Can the locations where documentation occurs house new EHR equipment? Are there space constraints to consider?
- ✔ Are you or your staff concerned about documenting on a computer in view of the patient?
- ✔ Will any roles require updated job descriptions to account for electronic documentation?
- ✔ What parts of documentation do staff feel will be easier to complete using the EHR? More difficult?
- ✔ Are there any patient scenarios that might be inappropriate for point-of-care (POC) documentation?
- ✔ What issues or questions must be resolved before medical staff is on board with the decision to use computers for documentation?

Table 8-1 gives you a start on documenting your visit workflows.

Table 8-1	Visit Documentation Roles and Responsibilities		
Role	**Responsibility**	**Location**	**Time of Documentation**
Physician			
Practitioner			
Nurse			
Medical Assistant			
Front Office			
Billing			

After visit communications

You need to chart your methods for handling any communications that occur after the patient has left your office. This is where you think about how you talk and work with your employees and colleagues to relay vital patient information.

✔ **Prescription refills**

- How do patients request a prescription refill?

- Who handles the call?

- How is the physician involved in the process?

- Can a nurse complete the refill for certain medications or patients without notifying the physician?

- How is the event documented in the paper chart?

✔ **Telephone calls**

- How many patient phone calls are received each day?

- Who handles phone messages and is there a triage process?

- How many of each kind of message are received each day (scheduling, emergency appointments, medical question, advice, billing issue, lab results)?

- How is the physician involved in the telephone call process?

- How do you manage after-hours calls?

- How is the event documented in the paper chart?

✔ **Lab and other study follow-up**

- How do you receive results for lab, radiology, and other studies?

- Does the physician review all results? If so, does he or she have the paper chart pulled at the same time?

- Who communicates results and findings to the patient? How is that communication documented?

- Do you send letters, call the patient, or some combination of the two depending on the results?

✔ **Referrals (incoming and outgoing)**

- What information is sent to the referred physician or practice? Who pulls that information together?

- How do you obtain preauthorization? How is that documented in the chart?

- What happens with the results from a patient referral? Does the physician sign off on each referral letter?

- Does the physician send a formal letter summarizing the patient encounter or encounters to the physician who referred a patient?

- Does the physician send a request for referral letter when referring a patient to another provider?

If you use any sort of e-mail system or Web site to communicate with patients (pre-EHR), then you can also note how those procedures work. Your new EHR will minimize the need to use several other electronic platforms, but thinking about how EHR might improve your online communication efforts couldn't hurt.

Managing documents

You may be surprised to find that the way your documentation flows through the office is more like a raging rapids than a lazy river. There isn't always a direct path between the person who does the documenting and the file room. Files are pulled for quick reference, documents fall out of folders, files are taken from exam room to office, and sometimes papers get misfiled or lost. It's no wonder that you and your team want to eliminate some of this chart chaos and put all the patient data in one user-friendly, easy-to-access location where there's little likelihood something is lost in the document management shuffle.

Document management lies at the heart of why you are converting to the EHR. Be prepared to give it the weight it deserves and take the time to properly assess your workflow in this area. Your EHR will help index, store, and manage scanned or faxed items electronically.

Think about the documents you and your team manage and store: intake materials, HIPAA forms, charts, coding sheets, superbills, diagnostic results, orders, referral sheets, and so on. Then try to answer the following questions to get an idea of how your document management workflows operate:

- ✔ Who is charged with managing medical records? Is there a dedicated records staff or does the office staff share in the responsibility?
- ✔ If you have more than one office, is this activity centralized or does each office manage its own medical records?
- ✔ How much time is spent filing each day?
- ✔ When does chart prep occur?
- ✔ How much time do you spend on chart prep each day?
- ✔ Are there days that have higher document volume than others?
- ✔ What kind of documents enter your practice?
- ✔ How many documents do you scan per day?
- ✔ How many documents do you envision scanning after your EHR is implemented?
- ✔ Should you devote specific resources to batch scanning?

✔ How do you plan to sort documents from the batches into patient records?

✔ What type of scanning equipment will be available?

✔ How many scanning workstations will be available?

Think about the documents in your practice and how they enter your practice office. Consider how your workflow will change using an EHR to manage these documents:

✔ **Diagnostic test results** will be interfaced to your EHR so you'll no longer need to manage these documents.

✔ **Referral requests** can be electronic, reducing the number of paper-based referral letters and consult letters that are sent and received.

✔ **Images** can be accessed electronically in some cases, but you may still need to store physical films, store CDs, or scan EKG strips.

✔ **Clinical summaries or discharge summaries** can be exchanged electronically using your EHR.

✔ **Paper documents** can be scanned and categorized using your EHR.

Identifying Opportunities for Process Improvement

When you know your practice's workflow design, you can plan your new workflows for after you implement the EHR. Consider this the "blue sky" portion of the workflow redesign process. In other words, the sky's the limit for thinking of more efficient ways to improve the quality of workflows and processes.

You can identify some of the areas for improvement by reviewing your answers to the questions you answered when evaluating your workflows and recognizing recurring themes or issues. For example, if you notice that many of your team members noted difficulties in relaying lab results to the primary physician in a timely fashion, you can prioritize making use of the EHR's instant messaging functions.

Understanding your pain points

You need to confirm what isn't working in your workflow model and where you have opportunities to improve. You may be experiencing workflow "pain" in such categories as the following:

✔ **Throughput:** Issues of timing or documenting patient flow in and out of the clinic.

✔ **Clinical outcomes:** Improved screenings or immunizations, for example.

✔ **Financial:** Reimbursements, documentation issues, charge capture, and so on.

The areas of operational redesign — patient flow, visit documentation, after visit communications, and document management — can help you organize your pain points to help you create a future workflow that maximizes the power of your EHR. Use the areas in conjunction with the goals and mission of your practice (see Chapter 4) and the analysis of your workflows to determine areas for improvement. You can also think about some general goals in each of those areas to help frame your discussion about improvement opportunities.

Overall goals

What you want the EHR to do for your practice in terms of patient flow can be directly related to your general clinical philosophy about patient care. Think of it like this: In an ideal world, how would you move patients through your practice each day while providing them with the most efficient and optimal care? Think about the following questions:

✔ Is improvement of patient and information flow one of the reasons that you're moving to an EHR?

✔ What specific issues or challenges do you think the EHR will help improve?

✔ What are the employees' fears or concerns about patient care as related to implementing the EHR?

✔ What EHR features does the team feel must be included to achieve more efficient patient flow?

With the patient flow picture fresh in your mind, think about your practice's specific mission and goals for each major portion of the patient flow process. Compile specifics for each of the following categories with some appropriate goals:

✔ **Check-in**

- Reduce the amount of redundant information that your staff collects from patients.

- Create automated tools for patients to enter and validate their own information.

✔ **Rooming patients**

- Integrate automated collection of patient vitals.

- Validate key patient information including medications, family history, and past medical and surgical histories.

✔ **Provider visit**

- Incorporate nursing- or patient-entered information into the physician note.

- Engage the patient in their care through the EHR's diagrams, trending graphs, and results review.

✔ **Check-out**

- Collect all appropriate fees prior to discharge.

- Facilitate follow-up appointments, referrals, and diagnostic study scheduling prior to the patient leaving the office.

✔ **Nurse visits**

- Create automated templates and protocols for quick visits.

- Automate physician notification and nurse visit sign-offs.

Use the information you gleaned when you took inventory of your practice workflows.

Visit documentation goals

Make your patient care tasks official by properly documenting them. After you have the EHR up and running, you'll find that many of the documentation responsibilities are shared throughout the practice (thank you, automated forms!). But for now, you're still living in a paper world.

Set up some documentation goals by thinking about how, exactly, the EHR is going to help you avoid some of the pitfalls you have experienced by reviewing and analyzing what you and your staff do on a given day. Here are some things to think about when you are setting documentation goals:

✔ What information needs to be documented in the presence of the patient and what can be documented in another location at another time?

✔ How can information entered by the nurse, medical assistant, or other care team member help the overall visit documentation?

✔ What are the benefits of performing POC documentation for the practice, provider, and patient?

✔ Do you think interaction between the provider and patient will improve when documentation uses a computer? How?

✔ Could the new documentation process negatively impact the office visit for the patient or the provider?

✔ How will the provider's office life improve if POC interactions are documented using the EHR?

✔ How can computerized documentation improve efficiency?

✔ What templates can be created to document standard visits or key clinical information?

✔ What visuals might the provider share with the patient such as changes in trends for lab values or vitals?

After visit communication goals

How you communicate with other office stakeholders regarding these important workflows is often directly related to your overall clinical philosophies. How well you and your staff relay information often reflects the state of the office environment. The EHR can't necessarily change the corporate communication culture, but it may open the door to a higher level of interoffice communication and improve how you share information and responsibilities. Think about the following questions:

✔ How should the EHR improve after visit workflows?

✔ What are the ideal scenarios according to the providers, office staff, and patient?

✔ Do those ideas differ? How?

✔ Are there specific communication issues you hope the EHR can address?

✔ What are the staff concerns about EHR and communication? Provider concerns?

After you answer some of these communication questions, you can set up some goals for how EHR implementation can inform your after visit workflows. Some categories and potential goals to consider include

✔ **Prescription refills**

  • Automate the request from the patient or pharmacy.

  • Provide easy workflow for the physician to automatically sign off on refills.

✔ **Telephone encounters and e-visits**

- Create workflow for nurse or physician to start a telephone encounter and easily route to other staff members for the completion of documentation.

- Identify opportunities to appropriately charge for telephone encounters or e-visits facilitated through your patient portal (discuss this with your insurance companies).

✔ **Test results**

- Automatically interface test ordering and test results into the EHR.

- Create templates to send patient letters regarding results.

- Populate a patient portal with appropriate result information.

✔ **Referrals**

- Create automatic outgoing referral templates with patient information that can be e-mailed, faxed, or mailed to other physicians.

- Automatically check to see whether a patient needs preauthorization prior to scheduling the referral.

Goals for managing paper

Compiling your goals for reducing paper charts is probably pretty high on your EHR to-do list. After all, one of the bonuses of implementing EHR is no longer having to deal with cumbersome paper documentation. You still have to document procedures, patient visit information, results, and referral information, though — as of now, the EHR does not offer ESP capabilities! Here are some questions to consider when you create your document management goals:

✔ Do you want to move paper charts offsite? If so, do you want any paper documents to remain onsite?

✔ How long do you need to keep your patient records in the office before moving them offsite? (If you didn't input all patient information via scanning or abstraction, you'll probably want to hold on to your paper records for a while.)

✔ Can you really create a "paperless" environment? What do you hope to gain from it?

✔ What do you want to change about any manual document processes?

✔ Are providers and staff members apprehensive about eliminating chart pulls for visits, phone calls, or follow-ups?

✔ How much time do you want to save in terms of document filing, refilling, and chart pull?

✔ How can you redeploy your staff since they won't be pulling charts? (Be mindful that your staff may be concerned about losing their jobs.)

✔ How will you handle the paper that still is sent to your office from outside labs, hospitals, other providers, and patients?

Planning for an EHR-Enabled Workflow

With so much information swimming in your head, imagining your new clinical life with an EHR is probably difficult. But, lucky for you, you have the services of your vendor rep at the ready and, if the vendor is worth its software, that rep will be happy to assist you with identifying opportunities for creating a future workflow.

This can be (if the vendor seizes the opportunity) a great chance for the rep to really show you what the EHR can do to improve workflows. With the sales phase (when the rep was focused on showing you the bells and whistles) over, he or she can really dig in and show you some of the less flashy, but useful, EHR features that can make life smoother for employees. Involve your vendor in the workflow redesign process so you can understand the functionality of the EHR on a larger level and get an outside viewpoint on ways to improve workflow design.

You can create any workflow redesign process you like. But, by and large, you can create your new workflow by following these steps:

1. **Identify opportunities to update workflows.**

   If some processes won't necessarily change from the EHR implementation, yet you want to improve them to allow them to gel with other processes that will change, make a point to develop some potential updates for them.

2. **Identify new workflow opportunities.**

   With the EHR implementation, processes that weren't possible before, such as connecting electronically and automatically to your regional health information exchange or local hospital, become possible. The establishment of new processes involves some trial and error, but that's why you are including your vendor rep in this process. It's safe to say this won't be his or her first rodeo — the rep has done this a time or two before, maybe hundreds of times. Rely on his or her expertise when establishing EHR-related workflows.

3. Map your potential new and improved workflows.

You can use your existing word processing or presentation software (like Word or PowerPoint) to create workflow maps or flowcharts to help you visualize your potential workflow updates. Or just plain old pen and paper works just fine, too. Your vendor might also recommend software you can use to create a customized workflow chart. Figure 8-3 shows a workflow chart.

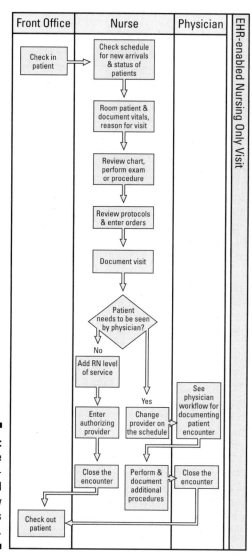

Figure 8-3:
A sample EHR-enabled workflow process map.

Don't worry — the flowcharts you create now aren't necessarily set in stone. You're identifying opportunities, not making final decisions about how your new workflows will operate.

Participating (Effectively and Efficiently) in the System's Design

You are a key participant in the design of your EHR system because you have a firm handle on how you want your workflow design to operate. The EHR is a vital element of your new workflow design, and vice versa. The two work together to provide your stakeholders with the best clinical care scenario possible. Therefore, be the workflow champion when it comes to designing and implementing your EHR.

System design

Armed with your list of goals and your new flowcharts, you can work with your vendor rep and other EHR transition team members to ensure that the new system will incorporate your newly designed workflows and help you provide the most efficient care. Dialogue openly with your vendor rep while you work together to design and test the specific functions of the EHR.

Work with your vendor and its team to design and customize the system to accommodate your needs and these new and improved workflows you've been considering. When using the EHR, you'll want to collect some information every time you and your staff document a patient encounter, yet limit choices at other times. The vendor can point out these options to help you make the right decision.

Additionally, you can customize certain "out of the box" templates from the vendor. Some of these are documentation templates for certain visit types; others might be common letters or referral guidelines. Ask the vendor to teach you how to customize their standard content and then divide those responsibilities between the appropriate clinicians in your practice.

Ask your vendor and colleagues from the same specialty if they have any documentation templates or order sets that they can share with you. No reason to reinvent the wheel if you don't have to. If you have no one to ask, see whether the vendor can connect you to someone or check with your specialty society. Regional Extension Centers (RECs) are also tasked with helping primary care providers with workflow redesign so your local REC likely has some resources for you as well.

When you test the EHR, run practice scenarios with your new workflow design to identify areas for improvement. You never truly know that a workflow functions correctly until you test it using the new software. Whether you are the guinea pig or you ask employees to test processes during office downtime, make sure someone documents the results of the testing and reports developments to the transition team and vendor rep.

Training

The new and improved workflows will prove to be a vital component of the training process. In addition to new workflow designs, employees will need to learn EHR processes and procedures. You and the transition team can work with your vendor rep to determine the most efficient way to relay both kinds of information to your staff.

Not everyone embraces change. If you position the new workflows as benefits, your employees are more likely to be on board when training occurs. Also, show participants the information you gathered about how long a process takes and how they'll save time by using the EHR.

After you can confirm that a new EHR workflow is successful, you can create related reference documentation and manuals to support and reinforce these processes. You may opt for a desk manual or an easy-to-access online document that details how to operate each process. Work with your transition team and employees to create the model that works best for you and then incorporate that information into your training documents.

Support

Keep support flowing for general EHR education and workflow design changes. You can remind everyone of their new workflows in all sorts of ways, from verbal reminders to document-based support materials. You may find it helpful to host regular meetings focused solely on reviewing and revising EHR-enabled workflows. When the staff gets the swing of the new model, you can offer support as needed.

Consider creating ongoing support documents that everyone can easily access. You can convert training materials into support materials or create "quick-reference" guides based on more detailed support materials.

Evaluate your new workflows after you go-live. Establish a period that will provide you enough time to really use the new systems and note how or if you would like to revise them.

Realizing improved benefits

Take time to evaluate the benefits of your EHR outcomes. Determine a time (say, a few months post go-live) when you can evaluate the outcomes of your new workflow design and address any areas for change or improvement. Make a few more lists (yep, more lists) and work with your transition team to note (and celebrate) the positive outcomes as well as discuss the areas you hope to improve. We talk more about system improvement and your workflows in Chapter 16.

Chapter 9

Assigning New Roles and Responsibilities

*B*y now, you know about all the great things an EHR can do for your practice and your patients. The availability of electronic patient information can make a lot of your practice's work easier. Entering and capturing the information will likely make some of your practice's work harder, at least in the beginning. The key to making this EHR transition bearable is understanding how roles and responsibilities change. New roles are created, certain jobs are modified, and (thankfully) some old archaic functions are no longer needed.

In this chapter, we help you understand the functions needed to effectively implement and use an EHR in your practice. With a little preparation (okay, sometimes it will be *a lot* of preparation), your physicians and staff will be happier in their new jobs!

Restructuring the Front Office

The front office is the central hub and nexus of your practice. Your staff is critical to efficient patient flow, ensuring good customer service, and financial success. The general functions of the front office, such as scheduling patients, reception, patient check-in, collecting insurance, processing payments, answering the phone, and preparing patient information for the physician or nurse, do not go away in the electronic world, but how each person does their job definitely changes. We think it's for the better — there's less searching for paper charts and pulling patient files, and improved electronic tools.

Don't make a mistake many practices do by neglecting the impact of EHR implementation on the front office and focusing only on the clinical documentation by physicians and nurses.

Because the patient's first interaction with your practice is with front office staff — whether in person or by telephone — it's critical to involve front office team members in the EHR implementation so they understand how their jobs will be affected. Table 9-1 shows the differences each job may have after you implement EHR.

Table 9-1	Old versus New Front Office Functions	
Function	*Before EHRs*	*After EHRs*
Capture insurance and ID information	Photocopying	Scanning
Prepare patient chart for patient encounter	Searching and pulling charts	Charts available; determine whether additional preloading or scanning is needed (initially)
Document patient telephone inquiry	Paper note or log, direct follow-up with physician or nurse	Document request electronically and assign to responsible provider
Transmit patient prescription to pharmacy	Fax to pharmacy at patient check-out	Capture preferred pharmacy information at patient check-in; physician transmits prescription electronically
Schedule follow-up appointments	Maintain paper logs to track needed or missed follow-up	Run reports to identify and contact patients that need to come in for follow-up visit
File results (lab, radiology) in patient chart	Notification of physician of faxed result; file result in chart	None — physician notified of result electronically
Notify patient of drug recall	No method to identify patients	Call patients based upon EHR report
Provide patient with copy of chart upon request	Photocopy pages	Send chart to printer or fax directly from EHR; enable patient access via patient portal
Determine patient eligibility (medical, prescription)	Telephone call to insurer or PBM	Automated eligibility checking

Preloading of Patient Charts

Imagine your front office with no more paper appointment books, filing cabinets, and chart stacks. With an EHR, you can reduce the size of your paper chart storage and eventually eliminate it! Your file room space can eventually be converted to additional workspace, another patient room, or larger patient waiting area.

Those very tall and very full filing systems in your practice contain extensive history on thousands of patients. To avoid navigating back and forth between the computer and paper chart, patient clinical information is preloaded into the EHR. *Preloading* is the process of entering relevant clinical information into the EHR before go-live. Preloading can contribute greatly to workflow efficiency:

✔ You have access to an electronic patient chart with relevant historical information available during the next office visit.

✔ Eliminates the need for shuffling between paper and the computer during the patient encounter.

✔ Prevents the impractical and time-consuming process of entering historical information during a very short 10- or 15-minute office visit.

✔ Triggering of clinical decision support rules (such as drug-drug, drug-allergy interaction checking) during the patient's additional visits.

Thinking about preloading all those charts can be very overwhelming. To get your entire practice through this process, stay focused and committed to the goals of having coded electronic data that enables decision support, eliminating paper charts, and never searching for a chart again. Reiterate these goals to your staff while they're going through the tedious preloading process. One of the added benefits of preloading patient information into the EHR is that the staff and physicians can get early exposure to the system, and this helps to augment formal training.

There is a variety of philosophies on preloading, and the following sections guide you through putting together the policies and procedures that are best for your practice.

Deciding what information to preload

There is no established rule or convention on how much patient history information you should preload into your EHR. You don't need to preload information from every patient who has ever visited your clinic and you also don't need to preload every piece of information from the paper chart.

Instead, focus on a critical subset of data to obtain a snapshot of the patient for decision support. Preloading all the information from all the patient charts housed in your practice is neither practical nor feasible.

Preload information only for your active patients. You have to determine which patients are considered "active" within your practice based upon specialty, patient population, and practice culture. General convention, particularly for primary care practices, is to preload charts for patients who

✔ Had an office visit within the last 18–24 months

✔ Have a scheduled appointment within the first month of go-live

✔ Are seen regularly by the practice because of chronic conditions

Consider preloading the following information for all active patients:

✔ Active problems, conditions, and diagnoses

✔ Active medications

✔ Active allergies and sensitivities

✔ Advanced directives

✔ Relevant family and social history

✔ Relevant procedures and treatments

✔ Prior hospitalizations, surgeries, and severe illness

For adult patients, include:

✔ Recent test and lab results

✔ Recent immunizations

✔ Most recent vitals (more if needed per policy)

For pediatric patients, include:

✔ All immunizations

✔ All heights, weights

✔ All head circumferences for patients under 3 years old

✔ All lengths for premature patients under 3 years old

At a minimum, preload problems, medications, and allergies information. Only relevant clinical data needs to be preloaded as structured and coded (where applicable) data. Review the Meaningful Use criteria as well to identify key information that should be documented in the EHR. For clinical information associated with a date, enter the original onset date, start date, or date noted in the paper chart.

For complex patients, such as patients who require frequent visits or have multiple chronic conditions, physicians can type or dictate (via voice recognition or transcription) a summary note or History of Present Illness (HPI) for the patient that consolidates the entire "patient's story" to supplement the entry of structured data.

Mark each preloaded patient chart with a sticker that displays the preload date and identifying information on the individuals that completed the preloading and review.

You probably don't want nonclinical staff entering sensitive information, such as problems, diagnoses, and past medical history that use coded values (such as ICD-9 codes). Instead, create a chart abstraction tool, a paper-based form that allows a clinician or staff member to abstract this information. This form provides an organized template for identification of the information to preload and can help nonclinical staff preload effectively.

We hear from physicians and practices who spend hundreds — and thousands — of hours preloading charts. Some of the practices are very happy that they preloaded their charts and could focus on an electronic workflow. Other physicians indicate that they didn't really understand the value of preloading and how to best enter patient data until they started using the system on a daily basis. Some of these physicians found themselves modifying their preloaded information after go-live and wished they had instituted a concurrent preloading process for the first few months after go-live. After you preload a few charts, test the data by going through a few mock patient visits. This helps you become proficient at using the EHR, reinforce the initial training you receive, and validate your preloading approach before your practice spends extensive hours preloading.

Scanning the rest of the patient's chart

You've identified key information, like problems, medications and allergies, that you'll preload into the EHR. But you want access to more past information such as key consults or visit notes, and you don't want to hand enter all that information, right? That's where scanning information can really help. The clear advantage in scanning patient charts is that all data for a patient is available from the EHR, and patient charts can be subsequently removed from the practice for offsite storage. Scanning the entire record is very labor-intensive and can take a lot of electronic storage space. However, the cost of electronic storage options gets less expensive each day. The important consideration for scanning is what to scan and when.

Information scanned into the EHR isn't structured or coded, so the EHR won't generate alerts based on this scanned information — but the chart is available at your fingertips. Actually, it's available at your fingertips if your scanning process includes manually entering descriptive information about each document and/or visit type and then associating the information with the patient in the EHR.

Some software solutions can generate barcode stickers with patient identification and document type information that you can affix to documents; you can then scan documents in batches and match this scanned info with the patient's chart in the EHR. Your EHR vendor may also offer this service.

If you can determine chronic disease or severely ill patients by querying your current practice management system for "reason for visit" or diagnosis code, pull those charts for preloading and scanning.

Most practices opt to identify documents for scanning after the system is live. For the first few weeks to two months after go-live, have your front office staff pull paper charts for scheduled patients as they did previously. During the office visit, providers may identify documents for the front office to scan, such as relevant EKGs, ultrasound scans, consult notes, and patient consent forms.

Deciding who should be involved

The process of preloading should be a team effort where everyone in the practice — physicians, nurses, medical assistants, and office staff — participate. Participation in preloading helps to familiarize everyone in the office with EHR functionality and navigation.

The preloading process should begin as soon as the system design, build, testing, and initial EHR training are complete. Six weeks prior to go-live is a good time to start. Remember that you don't need to finish all of your charts prior to go-live. You will continue preloading after the go-live for patients that have upcoming visits.

Your practice will need to develop a policy that defines the schedule and amount of preloading for each role. Start with just a few trusted staff members, establish a review system and signature policy, and then add staff as you go:

   ✔ **Physicians, physician assistants, nurses, and nurse practitioners:** Initiate the preload process with this staff, set a daily benchmark of a few charts, and set the policies for coding and consistency of preloaded data. You don't want physicians preloading all of their patients, but try to have them preload 15 to 30 patients so your physicians learn how the EHR works.

✔ **Nonclinical staff, such as medical assistants and front-office personnel:** After you establish policies, nonclinical staff can preload data and ensure the review system you set up continues.

✔ **Temporary staff:** You may need to hire temporary staff to finish preloading data. Temporary and outsourced staffing firms offer resources specifically for preloading. Your EHR vendor may also provide some assistance and resources for this task.

Local medical students and nursing students are low-cost resources to assist with preloading, too.

Be sure staff is supervised and properly trained in your policies. If your practice opts to scan all or part of the patient chart, these temporary or nonclinical resources can scan charts of patients that already have structured preload data within the EHR.

During this process, your team will encounter important questions that provide an opportunity to set policies for standardization and consistency of preloaded data, especially coded data.

Deciding when to stop pulling charts

Approximately two weeks prior to go-live, the preloading workflow should shift focus to the patient appointment schedule for the first few weeks of go-live. Because preloading starts before go-live, information generated between the preload and the go-live will need to be entered in the paper chart and the EHR. For example, if a patient has an office visit or medication change/refill between the preloading of that patient's chart and the EHR go-live, the information will reside in the patient's paper chart, but you also need to enter the updated information into the EHR.

Undoubtedly, there will be patient visits during and soon after go-live for which data has not been preloaded into the EHR. Set a policy to determine whether the physician will enter this information during the encounter (which affects productivity) or the chart will be preloaded immediately before or after the encounter.

When you go-live, the front office staff will still pull the paper charts for each scheduled patient. This is often referred to as the *hybrid period*. In about 2–6 months after go-live, physicians should notice that preload information is available for the majority of patients and that clinicians are no longer referencing the patient chart for the majority of patient encounters. Another approach is to pull charts for the first 2–3 visits for a patient after EHR go-live.

Keep patient charts in your file room for 6–12 months or until your practice is only pulling charts on an ad hoc basis. At this point, you're ready to move those charts from the file storage area if that's your goal. Most practices send their paper charts to an offsite storage facility that will pull and deliver needed records on a regular schedule. You still have access to those charts, just not immediately, so agreeing with the decision to move the charts offsite is important for your practice. When determining your offsite storage needs, be sure to review your state's storage requirements for legal medical records. If you've scanned the entire record, check your state's requirements for whether you still need to hold on to that paper chart.

Processing What's Still on Paper

You are moving toward a *paperless* practice, not a practice with no paper. You'll still need to scan, fax, or print some documents. Don't worry, it's nothing compared to those paper charts that will soon be a distant memory.

Scanning after go-live

You still collect information that can't be generated or collected electronically that is scanned into the EHR outside the preloading process. For example, your practice may have photocopies of insurance cards that you'll need to scan. Patient registration and patient history information is largely captured via paper and then scanned. You may also need to scan reports or results that patients bring with them from another physician office or hospital. The number of practices implementing electronic kiosks, digital pen systems, and various data recognition technologies are limited at this time, but increasing. Until then, plan to scan some paper.

If you're interested in reducing the amount of patient intake documents you're scanning, ask your EHR or scanning vendor whether it supports the following data recognition technologies:

- **Optical Mark Recognition (OMR):** Reads optical marks (such as check marks) on a form, which could assist in capturing patient histories.

- **Optical Character Recognition (OCR):** Reads machine-written characters and letters, which could help determine paper document types and automatically match scanned documents with a patient's record and encounter.

- **Intelligent Character Recognition (ICR):** Reads written information, which could assist in collecting patient registration and history information.

Figure 9-1 shows how an OCR/ICR process works.

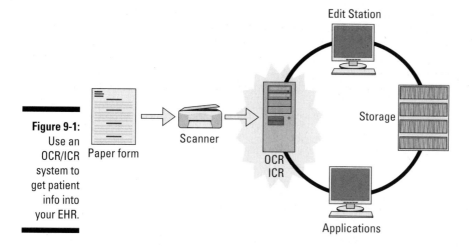

Figure 9-1: Use an OCR/ICR system to get patient info into your EHR.

Consult reports, lab results, radiology results, EKGs, letters, hospital/emergency department discharge summaries, procedure results, and other patient information will continue to arrive at your practice via mail or fax. Front office responsibilities will shift from placing these items into the paper chart to scanning the documents into the patient's EHR record. Each scanned document needs a corresponding document type within the EHR. This enables you to browse and view documents by type rather than searching one big bucket of scanned documents. In most cases, the patient (or the provider responsible for the patient) may need to be notified of receipt of these items.

When putting together your scanning policies and procedures, consider the following:

- ✔ What will be scanned? Are naming conventions and metadata setup in the EHR for each document type?

- ✔ Who will scan documents?

- ✔ When will scanning occur?

- ✔ Where will scanning occur? Will there be a dedicated workstation for scanning?

- ✔ How will documents be scanned? Batched at the end of the day? During the day?

- ✔ What is the volume of scanned documents? Is your scanner speed or system performance sufficient to support this volume? Do you have enough scanners? Do you have enough electronic file storage?

- ✔ Who needs to be notified of the scanned document (if applicable)? How will notification occur?

- ✔ What is the retention policy for the original or faxed hardcopy document?

Don't underestimate the time and resources that scanning documents requires. Set what you believe are reasonable goals based on your preloading experience. Monitor the amount of time and resources the scanning process takes during preloading and go-live. Assign individuals responsible for quality assurance (QA) — the validity and accuracy of scanned documents. If there's a scanning backlog, negative impact to practice workflow, or high error rate, you need to reevaluate and modify your scanning policies.

Faxing

Faxing documents generated within your practice's EHR should be much easier than in the paper environment. The ability to fax EHR information directly to other providers is built into most EHR solutions. You may need to set up a fax modem to enable this, so make sure your vendor covers this in your training session.

You can route inbound faxes to your practice to an inbound fax list within the EHR. Designate someone to monitor faxes received while the practice is open. From the received faxes list, the EHR can associate faxed documents with a patient's record and document type.

Your practice will continue to receive faxed renewal requests for prescriptions, but this should significantly decrease because of the electronic prescribing (e-prescribing) within the EHR. We provide guidance on managing faxed renewal requests later in this chapter.

Your practice may receive faxed lab results from labs your EHR doesn't interface with. To enable decision support, you have to enter the lab test and result values into the EHR. If you decide to enter these faxed results as structured data into the EHR, have a nurse perform this task with appropriate physician review.

Printing

With an EHR, your practice needs a printing policy. The majority of EHR workflows are streamlined within the EHR, but you'll need to print certain documents, such as patient instructions, medication lists, controlled substances prescriptions, and others. Do you want the physician to print documents for the patient from within the exam room to have the documents available to discuss with the patient? If so, a printer is required in each exam room. Other practices place printers in centralized locations where patients can be handed their paper-based information by front office staff or the provider at check-out. Make sure to review these workflows prior to your go-live.

Getting the Patient In and Out of the Office

An EHR should help your front office staff be more efficient and provide patients a certain level of service. Many of the functions performed by the front office to prepare, initiate, and complete the office visit will still occur, but these functions will be accomplished differently — and more easily — using the EHR.

Patient arrival and check-in

At the beginning or end of the day in the paper-chart world, your front office staff refiles patient charts from recent visits and checks the schedule to pull charts for the next day's visits. This file room back-and-forth will no longer be required soon after the go-live!

When the patient arrives to check-in for his or her appointment, you enter the patient arrival time and change the patient's status to indicate the patient has arrived. In most EHRs, arriving the patient within the system can generate notifications or triggers for clinical staff (medical assistant, nurse, and physician) that the patient has arrived and is in the waiting room.

Front office staff can verify address and insurance information, collect new information if necessary, and initiate electronic medical eligibility checking to verify eligibility and determine co-pay amounts. This means no more long phone calls for verification of coverage.

 Because your front office staff can quickly determine the co-pay, have them collect payment when the patient checks in. Prior to EHRs with electronic eligibility determination, practices often had extended accounts receivable periods because of patients forgetting to stop by the check-out desk to pay after their visit.

Most practices provide patients with a printout of demographic and past medical history information, as well as consent and HIPAA forms. A patient can then review this information and indicate whether any information has changed. Some practices may implement some of the data recognition technologies or utilize kiosks in the waiting room, but the most common approach is an intake form that includes EHR information.

Scan the patient consent and HIPAA forms into the EHR. The front office should verify that the status of any consent forms is visible within the EHR and update the patient's status accordingly.

Collect and verify the patient's preferred pharmacy information at check-in so the physician can electronically prescribe any needed prescriptions during the visit with the patient.

The EHR gives you the ability to view all prior or outstanding orders that were placed during or since the last visit. The front office can review any test orders and determine whether results are in the patient's electronic chart. If results aren't in the patient's chart, the front office staff can assist in locating them.

When the medical assistant or nurse is ready to take the patient into a patient room, the patient location and/or room number should be updated in the EHR to let the physician know that the patient is waiting in the room.

Checking out

The integrated coding and billing within the EHR eliminates the need for the superbill and encounter form when the patient is ready to leave. The check-out desk should know the details of the visit, verify any charges or payments, and provide any necessary next steps — whether that's scheduling another appointment, setting up tests, or referring the patient to another provider. Print any orders, prescriptions, or referral letters initiated by the physician and hand them to the patient.

Communicating test results

Implementing ordering and results interfaces can greatly reduce the administrative overhead that the front office bears from frequent faxing. The constant monitoring of the fax machine, organizing the results with patient charts, and notifying the physician will no longer be necessary. With an EHR

- ✔ Lab and radiology results are automatically matched with the electronic patient chart if the interface is built to and from those ancillary systems.

- ✔ Lab results (adhering to lab terminology standards such as LOINC) are coded and available as structured, discrete data within the EHR.

- ✔ Results are sent to a provider work list or notification list indicating that review and signature is needed.

- ✔ Abnormal results are flagged within the system.

- ✔ Reports can be set up to view pending orders so that front office staff can easily determine the tests that require follow-up.

A new workflow for front office staff and nurses is needed to monitor interfaced results and initiate follow-up with physicians, but the workflow is driven by the EHR, not the fax inbox.

Your practice may want to consider developing a policy for communicating test results to patients. Some practices allow front office staff, medical assistants, or nurses to communicate normal results to patients.

Results and other patient communications that are not interfaced electronically will continue to arrive via fax or mail. For faxed results, your EHR's fax server will receive the fax in an electronic inbox that needs to be monitored by practice staff. The faxed result or document will need to be associated with a patient within the system and routed to a provider for review and signature. Faxed information is not coded within the EHR, so you need to prescribe that staff enter coded values into the EHR manually as part of the routing process to the physician. In-office lab tests that don't interface with the EHR need to follow this workflow, too.

Handling telephone inquiries and phone notes

The EHR can document telephone inquiries and route them to the appropriate individual. There's also a priority flag to mark urgent inquiries. With an EHR, the person answering the phone has immediate access to the patient chart and may be able to respond to the question or document the inquiry in a more useful manner for the provider. You can also document the telephone encounter as a phone note within the EHR.

Appointment reminders

If your practice has a scheduling system, your office staff is likely already calling patients to remind them of upcoming visits. Most EHRs allow you to set a reminder or flag for a follow-up appointment during an office visit. Additionally, if you want to see a patient, you can set a reminder or notification for office staff to schedule an appointment. Some EHRs can also send a message to the patient either through standard mail or through a patient portal. The EHR can generate a list of patients who need to be seen (or are past due) but don't have a scheduled appointment. Therefore, if a patient leaves the office without setting up a future appointment, you have several ways to follow-up.

Charting the Patient Visit

The preceding sections of this chapter have predominantly addressed new functions for the office staff. This section presents a few new functions for the clinical staff to improve efficiencies and workflows via the EHR.

Most paper documentation tends to be top-to-bottom. Your practice may use paper documentation templates or chart covers that provide ways to organize and section key patient information in different areas of the chart, such as vitals, chief complaint/reason for visit, medications, and so on. Paper documentation is a static view of patient information in the exact way it was written.

With an EHR, the way you enter data is often not the way you view the data. Your practice can have electronic forms or views based on role or stage of the visit. When designing and implementing your EHR, you should consider the optimal view of information for a particular role or stage of the visit.

Intake/rooming the patient

After the front office indicates the patient has arrived and checked in, a medical assistant or nurse often initiates the intake process, rooms the patient, and updates the patient's location status in the EHR.

Because an EHR changes practice workflows, you have an opportunity to optimize them. You can now delegate work that doesn't require a physician's license. Your practice can have individuals operate at the highest level of scope of practice for their position.

In addition to measuring and documenting height, weight, and vitals, the nurse can also review and document the patient's medical history, document the reason for the visit, and perform an initial reconciliation of medications. Based on the reason for the visit or the problem/diagnosis list, the nurse likely has an opportunity to assist in preparing the patient for the physician. For example, if the diagnosis list indicates the patient has diabetes, the nurse may instruct the patient to remove his or her shoes and socks in anticipation of a diabetic foot exam.

Documenting the visit

Concurrent access to a patient's record using an EHR enables a physician to view a patient's information while the nurse or medical assistant is still rooming the patient. You can view records for your scheduled patients (and unscheduled patients) any time and any place you can access the Internet (for Web-based applications).

In the paper world, you'd have to flip through multiple sheets of paper to get a sense of your patient's progress or status. An EHR allows you to navigate past encounters and cycle through prior documentation sections, such as HPI documentation. This may be useful to you when you have a patient in for a follow-up and you want to view history or pull documentation from a prior visit.

Your EHR includes a flowsheet view of certain structured data, such as vitals and common labs results. If you want to see a common grouping of information for a particular diagnosis or visit type, work with your EHR vendor to set up default views. Figure 9-2 shows a sample diabetes management flowsheet.

Patient Name_____Birth Date__/__/__ Gender M__F__

PAYER & PATIENT NUMBER: CLINIC & PROVIDER:

Medicare_____   Clinic _____

Medicaid _____   Location _____

Other, please specify_____   Physician _____UPIN _____

ONGOING CLINICAL MEASURES

	Initial Measurement		Subsequent Measurements					
	Date mm/dd/yyyy	Results	Date mm/dd/yyyy	Results	Date mm/dd/yyyy	Results	Date mm/dd/yyyy	Results
LABORATORY								
Hemoglobin A1c *At Least Annual*								
FASTING LIPID PROFILE								
Total Cholesterol *Annual*								
HDL Cholesterol *Annual*								
LDL Cholesterol *Annual*								
Fasting Triglycerides *Annual*								
Urinalysis for protein *Annual*		Pos Neg		Pos Neg		Pos Neg		Pos Neg
Quantitative/Semi-Quantitative Urine Protein*		Pos Neg		Pos Neg		Pos Neg		Pos Neg
Microalbumin**								
Creatinine *Annual*								
MONITORING	Date	Results	Date	Results	Date	Results	Date	Results
Diabetic Foot Exam *Annual*								
Dilated Eye Exam *Annual*								
Blood Pressure *Each Visit*								
Weight *Each Visit*								
Review Home Blood Glucose Monitoring *Each Visit*		Yes No		Yes No		Yes No		Yes No
PREVENTIVE CARE	Date	Results	Date	Results	Date	Results	Date	Results
Influenza Vaccination *Annual*		■		■		■		■
Pneumococcal Vaccination								
Tobacco Counseling *PRN*		Nonsmoker Yes No		Nonsmoker Yes No		Nonsmoker Yes No		Nonsmoker Yes No
Diabetes Education *Each Visit*		Yes No		Yes No		Yes No		Yes No
Dietary Instruction *Each Visit*		Yes No		Yes No		Yes No		Yes No

Figure 9-2: A sample diabetes flowsheet.

Set up your EHR to provide automatic reminders in the exam room for when a patient is due for preventive or disease management services. This can be helpful when a patient is in your office for a reason other than disease follow-up or preventative care, but still past due for a test, procedure, or evaluation.

Generating prescriptions, orders, referral letters, school/work letters, and so on can be more efficient with an EHR. Many EHRs offer links — to within the EHR and to Internet sites — to patient education materials. Because you usually need to provide the patient with printed copies or summaries of these items, equipping each exam room with a printer is ideal. If your exam room size or layout prohibits a printer in each exam room, place a printer as close to the exam room as possible. Printers placed outside the exam room cause physicians to leave the room multiple times, which might contribute to patient frustration and extend the duration of the encounter beyond the scheduled visit slot.

Ironically, research shows that EHRs cause some clinicians to engage less with patients because, relative to paper charts, so much more information is available before actually seeing the patient. Getting used to new workflows and all the information accessible to you can take some time.

EHRs also offer links to evidence-based guidelines for diagnosing and treating specific conditions. The patient education and evidence-based guidelines accessible within the EHR can be helpful tools in engaging patients in their care and communicating your medical decisions.

Your EHR can help you generate the following information to engage and educate patients:

- ✔ **Reconciled medication list:** Print a copy of the patient's reconciled medication list and review it with the patient. This medication list should communicate previous medications, added medications, and all active medications for review with the patient.

- ✔ **Copy of e-prescription, e-orders, or e-referrals:** Print a confirmation or copy of the electronic prescription so patients know the prescription has been sent to their preferred pharmacy. Printing a confirmation of electronic lab orders and referrals for the patient can serve as a useful reminder, too.

- ✔ **Patient education or instructions:** Print a copy of the patient education materials and review them with the patient.

- ✔ **Paper orders or referrals:** Not all orders or referrals can be sent electronically, but the EHR can track orders and generate the paper requisition or referral for the patient.

- ✔ **School notes and work letters:** Generate these easily within the EHR and provide them to the patient.

Ideally, you won't print all of this information separately. Most EHRs allow you to print an After Visit Summary that contains the list of reconciled medications, all new orders, follow-up visit information, and patient instructions. The physician or nurse can take the time to review this summary with the patient prior to his departure to confirm he understands exactly what the plan is.

Managing Prescription Renewal Requests and E-Prescriptions

In 2004, the Medical Group Management Association (MGMA) determined that the administrative complexity related to managing prescription refill requests just by phone could cost practices more than $10,000 per year per physician. That's a lot of dough, even for a large multi-physician practice. Thanks to your shiny new EHR, though, you can reduce costs and time spent calling in scripts.

Sending prescriptions electronically reduces paper flow and gives your fax machine a needed rest. An EHR-based e-prescription system allows you and your staff to consider possible medications for a patient within the context of patient history, diagnoses, recurring illnesses or problems, test results, and any drug allergies or interaction issues. Additionally, workflow improves because of greater accessibility for your office staff, particularly when a physician is out of the office or inaccessible for patient questions. Other benefits of e-prescriptions include

- ✔ Enhanced patient safety (reduced errors, fewer drug interaction issues)
- ✔ Improved patient medication compliance
- ✔ Better prescription accuracy and efficiency
- ✔ Reduced healthcare costs

Informing your most-used pharmacies that you're switching to e-prescribing is a great reason to touch base about any other questions or concerns they (or you) may have about EHR adoption in general. It's a good time to ask some anecdotal information about their experience with the process.

Informing your patients of your office's new e-prescription system is vital, too. Because you'll inform them of your overall EHR plan, this can be a component of the same patient education. Make the education process very customer service–oriented and focus the discussion on each individual patient's needs and how they'll be addressed with e-scripts. In other words, if you make it personal, your patients are more likely to be on board. For example, your patients will no longer leave your practice with a hardcopy prescription, so it's helpful to provide them with a medication list or confirmation that medications have been e-prescribed.

Unfortunately, EHR vendors provide little in the way of e-prescribing training as a part of your overall EHR training. So, be sure to communicate specific questions to your vendor to get the most complete answers for you and your staff. Some potential training questions to ask might include the following:

- ✔ How can I find a specific medication in the database?

- ✔ What do I do if I can't find the medication I am looking for?

- ✔ How do I handle special prescription situations like pediatric dosing and prescribing medical supplies?

- ✔ How do I write a script for a compound medication?

- ✔ Why isn't a particular pharmacy in my system? How do I get it in my system?

- ✔ What do specific error messages mean? How do I overcome them?

- ✔ Can I write a prescription directly from a patient history screen?

You can find these and other useful questions to ask in "A Clinician's Guide to Electronic Prescribing" — a useful document developed by the eHealth Initiative (www.ehealthinitiative.org) and the Center for Improving Medication Management that details many of the most commonly asked questions about planning and implementing e-prescribing.

Ask your EHR vendor whether she provides online tutorials, presentations, or webinars geared to e-prescribing training, especially if the vendor doesn't provide much hands-on training.

Wondering why you are receiving faxed or phone renewal requests? Here are a few reasons and recommendations to help get your e-prescribing renewals workflow out of the dark ages:

- ✔ **Was the prescription initially sent electronically?** If the prescription wasn't prescribed electronically (say it was entered into the EHR, but was printed or transmitted via fax), the renewal request can't be electronic.

- ✔ **Is it for a controlled substance?** Until recently, controlled substances could not be prescribed electronically. The dual workflow of sending some prescriptions electronically and others via paper can be disruptive, not to mention confusing to patients. Now you can prescribe controlled substances electronically if you are eligible and both your EHR and receiving pharmacy systems follow the required guidance (see the nearby "E-prescribing of controlled substances" sidebar).

- ✔ **Was the medication prescribed by a provider in your office that is no longer working there or out of the office?** If a renewal request is routed to a provider that is no longer active in your practice, or the order results in an error, the renewal request is going to come in as a fax.

- ✔ **Did the patient call the practice instead of the pharmacy to request the renewal?** Encourage your patients to call their pharmacy to request renewals instead of the office. That way, the pharmacy initiates the electronic renewal request, and the EHR links the prescription to the patient's chart and the medication list for you.

E-prescribing of controlled substances

Electronic prescribing of schedules II through V controlled substances is allowed in the United States. The Drug Enforcement Administration (DEA) released its Interim Final Rule in March 2010 (effective June 1, 2010) on e-prescribing controlled substances, requiring two-factor authentication. You need two different and independent methods for the EHR to authenticate you — that is, verify that you are who you say you are. You can do this a few ways (and more technologies are emerging): unique passwords, biometrics (fingerprint scan, iris scan, voice scan), and devices (hardware tokens, smart cards, PIN numbers via SMS using a cell phone).

Here's the hard part: You have to be using a "compliant application" that can handle the direction provided in the Interim Final Rule. Because the requirement was just established in March 2010, many EHRs and pharmacy systems haven't been updated to handle this, and software updates could take up to 18 months. Also, some vendors are likely waiting for additional clarifications to the Final Rule prior to finalizing their software and making it available for general release.

Talk to your vendor and consult your professional organization for additional guidance about electronic prescribing of controlled substances. For example, the American Medical Association (AMA) provides a summary of the DEA's Interim Final Rule on Controlled Substance E-Prescribing at www.ama-assn.org.

Consider tasking electronic renewal requests to one person on your staff — such as a physician assistant or nurse practitioner — to help streamline workflow.

For renewal requests that come in via fax, your front office can enter them into the EHR and task a provider to renew them electronically.

Maintaining and Monitoring with the EHR

The EHR, as cool as it is, doesn't operate in a vacuum, and it's definitely not HAL from *2001: A Space Odyssey*. You and your staff are the brains of this operation, so you have to make the EHR work for you. As the point person for the adoption, you need to facilitate the maintenance and monitoring of the program to ensure it works to its fullest potential for your practice. You can do this by creating a daily task list, communicating with others in the office, keeping an eye on billing accuracy and claims, and changing practice operations based on EHR quality reports.

Creating task lists

What needs to happen for your patients today? Answer that million-dollar question and you have a task list. Each day, you can create a task in the EHR that covers both individual tasks and reactive tasks for you, your colleagues, and your staff. These tasks fall into the "Things I Need to Do or Plan Based on What I Think Will Happen Today" category, such as planning for incoming patients, outreach, and reporting; or the "Things I Need to Do to Follow Up on Previous Patient Interactions" category, such as creating notes, lab follow-ups, and prescriptions. Most EHRs can also generate a patient-specific task item or alert to set a reminder for the next time you see the patient — something like, "Things to Ask the Patient during the Next Visit".

Communicating with others in your practice

The EHR can create an atmosphere of more open communication, so make use of the interactive functions it offers. Use the EHR to send notes or reports to other providers, communicate go-forwards to the front office, and send alerts or reminders about incoming patients or necessary follow-up measures. In other words, save a lot of time on the phone and time wandering the halls of your office trying to find a staffer or colleague by using the EHR's message and alert features. For example, staff can pose questions to the physicians via the EHR's instant messaging (IM) function, rather than opening the exam room door and interrupting a patient consultation, which can be less intrusive and more time efficient.

Don't let the EHR be your excuse for not interacting with staffers and fellow colleagues. Maintaining personal and professional relationships via face-to-face interaction is vital to the health of your corporate culture. So, go ahead and chat it up around the conference table or water cooler.

Additionally, think about how everyone in the office manages patients — individuals and groups. The EHR allows you to create functions and tools designed to monitor not only individuals, but also categories of patients. You can use the EHR's support tools to create reminders for specific care tasks, follow-ups, and communication suggestions. For example, say that Mr. Jones is a patient with type 2 diabetes. The EHR can remind the front office staff to set up eye and foot exam appointments for him. Now, think about all the type 2 diabetes patients in your practice. The EHR can remind all intake staff to provide these patients with the most recent education handouts to help them manage their condition, not to mention adhere to best practice care guidelines. The EHR can look out for your office's communication needs, as long as you tell it to do so.

Improving billing accuracy and claims

You already know that implementing your EHR will save you time in the end; however, an EHR can also affect profitability by improving billing and claims accuracy. How you manage the EHR has a lot to do with ensuring those improvements.

Some EHRs base their functions on collections and billing analysis. If you want to make sure you and your staff improve in those areas and are interested in having the EHR help you do this, ask your vendor about how your new e-toy can maximize that focus.

Coding is the key to making sure your EHR is actually helping you improve in these areas. Your EHR will most likely offer drop-down lists of codes for the purpose of recording patient visits. This saves your staff from chasing down the right codes, but it can also become rote and disallow individual alterations based on specific patient needs. For example, if a patient presents with a skin condition that may have symptoms not typically associated with a skin disorder, the EHR may not prompt you or your staff to mark it, thus missing an opportunity for accurate coding. This could then affect the final billing or claim. You have to educate staff on ways to overcome this obstacle. Ask your vendor to provide training.

Although the EHR offers prompts, reminders, and drop-down lists a-plenty, the coding team members are professionally trained to keep up with the ever-changing landscape of coding rules and regulations that will keep your office in the black and in compliance.

Developing Quality Reporting that's Valuable for You and Your Patients

Quality reporting is something you were doing before, but probably not as efficiently. If you set up your EHR software to do so, you can create reports on just about every aspect of patient care quality.

Sometimes in the paper world, documenting everything in a patient discussion isn't easy. With EHR, check boxes and other functions make that documentation easier, and other systems allow you to pull info into physician notes to create reports that capture issues you wish to document.

When thinking about how you to set up quality reporting functions, consider what is important to your practice in relation to your patient client base. To get that $40,000–$64,000 available via the American Recovery and Reinvestment Act (ARRA), you have to demonstrate that you're using the EHR in a meaningful way that improves quality.

Some of the questions you should ask include the following:

- ✔ What are the components or characteristics of quality?

- ✔ What can be captured in an EHR? How can it be captured?

- ✔ What variables would cause the project to succeed or fail? How can we measure success?

- ✔ Do the quality measures have credibility?

- ✔ What will the electronic health data record support? Are the measures responsive to the changes that will be in place, such as computerized clinical decision support?

- ✔ Will the information change or modify treatment? Is the change significant?

- ✔ How reliable is the data? How easy is it to capture? In what form will it be captured?

- ✔ What are we going to measure? How are we going to measure it? How will we capture that in the routine flow of the clinical process?

Your office team plays an integral role in deciding how you want to set up quality reporting. Ask for their input on what patient information is most vital to quality reporting and have them assist in data collection in a way that complements how they already function in their roles.

Share your quality reports with staff and colleagues. Doing so puts a face on what they do each day and can empower them in their team roles.

Many EHRs either include or connect to quality reporting software that you can customize based on what you and your staff want to monitor. If the vendor's EHR doesn't provide this functionality, make sure to ask them for recommendations of software that integrates with their system.

These types of reporting tools are databases of clinical rules, which often change at a moment's notice. Using such a quality tool beats memorizing and keeping track of rules on an ongoing basis, and the database is updated with the latest new information. Clinical guidelines, protocols, pay-for-performance initiatives, and formulary and Meaningful Use requirements are often accessible through these tools. Setting up quality reporting can help you

- ✔ Access information about drug interactions and allergies
- ✔ Fulfill payment criteria
- ✔ Flag possible billing errors
- ✔ Participate in incentive programs
- ✔ Monitor reimbursement quality and frequency
- ✔ Interact with and respond to federal mandates and programs

---

Creating a quality report system

An article in the journal *Practice Management* titled "Beyond Charting: Using Your EHR's Data to Improve Quality" showcases one clinic's experience with quality reporting. They recommend some useful steps for setting up your own quality reporting system:

- ✔ Establish benchmarks
- ✔ Select champions
- ✔ Set goals for improvement
- ✔ Design and run reports

- ✔ Educate and communicate results to providers, staff, and patients
- ✔ Develop incentives
- ✔ Monitor results

Of course, it's up to you to create an atmosphere of quality control and a practice environment that embraces reporting. These general guidelines can be great discussion starters when you coordinate a quality plan with your team.

Chapter 10

Considering Security and Privacy

*T*he world is getting smaller in terms of information and who can access it. The advent of social networking sites, microblogs, and personal Web sites has increased everyone's visibility — even if they don't prefer the raised awareness. These days, it's no wonder that everyone is a little jittery about the security of their personal information, particularly their personal health record information.

Your clinic's new EHR may offer multiple points of access to patients' private health information (PHI), but that doesn't mean that every Joe with an Internet connection can surf your virtual file cabinet. Enter you, the EHR champion. One of your duties is to make sure that your EHR is secure, private, and accessible by only trusted stakeholders who provide care to your patients. Consider yourself the bouncer of this party — if someone misuses the EHR or gains unauthorized access to patient information, they're outta here! You also need to reassure patients and colleagues who have valid concerns about privacy and security.

Security and privacy add to the overall value of your EHR by increasing cost effectiveness, maintaining system reliability, and securing your reputation as a trusted champion for quality and security. In this chapter, you find out how you can make your EHR the most secure system on the block.

Understanding Security, Privacy, and Confidentiality

Who isn't concerned with information security these days? It seems that everyone has privacy on the brain concerning information — financial, personal, and even medical. No one wants their private healthcare information getting into the wrong hands.

Three areas to think about when it comes to the issue of sensitive patient health information are

✔ **Security:** The physical safeguards put in place to secure your patient's personal information

✔ **Privacy:** The patient's right to control the dissemination of his or her information

✔ **Confidentiality:** Who can access this sensitive information and for what reason

Figure 10-1 shows how these three concepts work together.

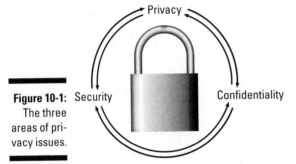

Figure 10-1: The three areas of privacy issues.

Security — Privacy — Confidentiality

To really understand the scope of security, privacy, and confidentiality in relation to your practice's EHR, you first have to put yourself in the shoes of your patients and consider EHR concerns from their point of view. In doing so, you may find that their apprehensions are your concerns as well. Some potential patient privacy concerns may include

✔ Who may view chart information (other physicians, lab techs, pharmacists, front office staff, and so on)

✔ How information is shared with other stakeholders

✔ What information, specifically, is part of the legal medical record

✔ What information is not part of the legal medical record but is still discoverable in a case

✔ How much other personal information (Social Security number, insurance ID number, names of relatives) is available electronically and to whom

✔ What, if any, outside entities may request electronic health information (potential employers or relatives, for example)

✔ How information is stored and backed up

✔ How old paper records are discarded or destroyed

✔ How record access history is recorded to assure that only appropriate staff is viewing files

✔ Who can run audit reports and what specific detail can the reports show

Your privacy and security measures take shape in two ways:

✔ Your practice's compliance with HIPAA lays the groundwork for promoting a clinical atmosphere that embraces the importance of securing patient information.

✔ The security of the EHR system keeps everyone's information private and accessible by only the people who need to see it in order to provide care.

The two concepts work together — by creating a secure environment, you also create a HIPAA-compliant one.

Security is not infallible, so there will always be some level of risk associated with sharing patient information. It might help you to think of security and privacy as two interrelated, living, breathing entities. Maintaining them both requires you to stay current on the latest trends and changes in technology and legislation that governs how you share patient information.

Keeping HIPAA Compliant

If you think there is no such thing as privacy anymore, you haven't read the Health Insurance Portability and Accountability Act (HIPAA) rules, specifically, the rules set for in Title II of HIPAA. These rules were established by the Department of Health and Human Services (HHS) to promote greater efficiency of information within the healthcare sector by tightening the security and privacy of personal healthcare data and establishing penalties for noncompliance.

If HIPAA compliance sounds über-serious, it is. You can bet your EHR budget that the fed doesn't mess around when it comes to the HIPAA rules and, as a result, has established some fairly clear-cut parameters to make sure that you cover all your practice's privacy bases.

Penalties for violating HIPAA regulations can include both civil and criminal penalties punishable by fines or imprisonment. Civil penalties can range from $100 to $50,000 per year for one violation. If someone is convicted of a criminal offense for disclosing or misusing personal health information, the fines may be substantial, ranging from $50,000 to $250,000 and one to ten years in prison.

HIPAA involves more than just having your patients fill out a form during the check-in process. This particular privacy act is big (the biggest, actually) and is one of the most far-reaching acts you experience while implementing the EHR.

HHS divides HIPAA into five categories of rules and standards that cover all your privacy bases: privacy, transactions and code sets, security, unique identifiers, and enforcement. In the following sections, we cover the privacy and security rules because they probably are at the top of your EHR-readiness to-do list. For more information about the specific details of HIPAA, visit www.hipaa.org.

If you are unsure whether HIPAA affects you, remember the acronym PCP: **P**lans, **C**learinghouses (like a billing service), and **P**roviders.

Privacy rule

Private health information (PHI) — a patient's health, care provisions, or associated payments — is protected by you, the covered entity. PHI is any information related to a patient, whether it is in print, in an electronic record, or even associated with a bill or payment history.

The privacy rule covers who *must* be notified of updates or additions to patient information and who *may* access the information. The "musts" are covered entities (that's you) that must report any PHI to the patient within 30 days of receiving a request to do so. You must also disclose PHI when required by law, for such instances as court cases or suspected child abuse.

The "mays" may disclose PHI in certain cases, as long as you make a reasonable effort to disclose only the minimum information necessary to get the job done. For example, if you receive a request from a colleague to obtain Mrs. Jones' latest mammogram results to facilitate treatment, that is all you should report. Her PHI about her latest bout of flu is not at issue, for example, and should not be disclosed in this case. So you, as covered entity, may disclose PHI for the following reasons:

- ✔ To facilitate treatment
- ✔ To initiate or follow up on payment
- ✔ To assist with healthcare operations
- ✔ If the patient has provided authorization to release the information

As resident EHR champion, you should make sure HIPAA's privacy rule is followed elsewhere within the practice. Many of those checks and balances happen via the EHR software, but it's a good idea to keep office dialogue open about how staffers and practitioners are understanding and implementing HIPAA regulations. Make sure you cover these vital privacy rule talking points:

- ✔ Patients have the right to ask you to rectify any incorrect PHI information.
- ✔ Patients have the right to be notified of how you use their PHI to provide or facilitate care. You must document each time you disclose information, what information you disclose, and how you communicate it.
- ✔ Patients have the right to confidential communication with anyone in your practice, and you are expected to make that happen. For example, if a patient asks that his or her health information be communicated only by mail, you must comply.

According to HIPAA legislation, your practice must appoint someone Privacy Official in charge of training employees and managing HIPAA complaints should they arise.

Security rule

Security is the other big ticket item on your HIPAA bill of goods. This rule works in conjunction with privacy, in that it covers similar information that exists in an electronic environment. Here's the breakdown: Privacy covers PHI in all its forms; whereas security covers information that exists only in e-form. Technically, the information covered by the security rule is known as Electronic Protected Health Information (EPHI).

Think of the security rule as a tiered set of requirements. The first tier includes three security categories within which your practice is required to comply: administrative, physical, and technical. Within those categories are specific security standards, some required and some suggested.

Administration requirements

Administrative safeguards cover how you create, manage, and disseminate information about your privacy procedures to employees, patients, and any governing agencies you answer to. To meet these standards, you have to create official written documents detailing your procedures, designate a privacy officer to manage privacy issues, and prove that your practice has management oversight for your policy structure, to name just a few.

Your policies must address certain key issues, such as

- Who within your practice will have access to EPHI

- How and why access is granted, modified, or terminated

- What sort of HIPAA initial and ongoing training is provided for employees

- How your practice will prove compliance on the part of third-party vendors (such as pharmacies, specialists and consultants)

- Emergency data backup and recovery plans

- Audit procedures for reviewing who accessed specific patient data (you decide which staff members will run audit reports and how often to audit)

Physical requirements

Physical safeguards are set up to help you control access to EPHI.

Physical requirements come into play during the implementation process; work with your vendor to set up controls that cover your hardware and software privacy needs.

These safeguards address

- Proper installation and disposal of hardware and software that does not compromise EPHI

- Who has access to equipment and software that might contain EPHI

- Overall security plans for your practice facility, records, and people who move in and out of your practice on a daily basis

- Workstation use, location, and security

- HIPAA training for third-party vendors who visit your office, such as technicians or maintenance personnel

Heeding HITECH and HIPAA

Although enforcing adherence to HIPAA can be difficult (you're cited for breaches only if *you* get caught), its cousin, the Health Information Technology for Economic and Clinical Health (HITECH) Act, imposes strict penalties for noncompliance.

HITECH extends the privacy and security rules of HIPAA to your practice's business associates. This means that any offending associates are also subject to civil and criminal penalties for noncompliance. Be sure to spread the word to anyone associated with your practice that they, too, are responsible for making HIPAA happen. HITECH imposes civil monetary penalties for violations of HIPAA by creating four categories of violations, each with enforcement provisions with increasing levels of severity and penalties:

✔ **Reasonable Diligence:** The offender did not know HIPAA was violated, and would not have known by exercising reasonable diligence: $100– $50,000 for each violation.

✔ **Reasonable Cause:** The violation is due to a reasonable cause, but not due to willful neglect: $1,000–$50,000 for each violation.

✔ **Willful Neglect, Timely Corrected:** The violation is due to willful neglect, but was corrected in a timely manner: $10,000– $50,000 for each violation.

✔ **Willful Neglect, Not Corrected:** The violation is due to willful neglect and was not corrected in a timely manner: $50,000 per violation up to $1,500.000 in a calendar year.

You can find out more on the Office of Civil Rights Health Information Privacy Web site at `www.hhs.gov/ocr/privacy/index.html`.

Technical requirements

Technical safeguards are set up to help you control access to your EHR and protect data you transmit from being intercepted by outside parties. These safeguards cover the following details:

✔ Protecting your EHR and other information systems from breach by using encryption, firewalls, and access controls

✔ Ensuring your practice doesn't allow unauthorized deletion or alteration to EPHI housed in its system

✔ Maintaining data integrity, thus ensuring that information is the same after it has been stored as it was when it was entered

✔ Authentication of third parties or outside entities; proving the outside parties are who they claim to be

✔ Documenting HIPAA practices and making them available to the government

✔ Inclusion of configuration settings in HIPAA documentation

✔ Risk analysis and risk management documentation

Making Your EHR Secure

Your EHR needs to be secure from the get-go. By working closely with your vendor rep, you can be sure the new system meets all the necessary HIPAA and HITECH privacy guidelines and protects your patients' information better than Fort Knox.

A secure EHR equals a profitable practice. By implementing security features with your EHR, you not only provide protection for your patients but also create a more cost-efficient system. If you're using an ONC-ATCB–certified EHR, many of the required privacy and security standards have been tested and verified as part of the certification process. Whew!

Here are a few of the security capabilities that are part of ONC-ATCB–certified EHRs:

- **Access control:** Assign a unique name and/or number for identifying and tracking user identity and establish controls that permit only authorized users to access electronic health information.

- **Emergency access:** Permit authorized users (who are authorized for emergency situations) to access electronic health information during an emergency.

- **Automatic log-off:** Terminate an electronic session after a predetermined time of inactivity.

- **Audit log:** Record actions related to electronic health information and enable a user to generate an audit log for a specific time period and to sort entries.

- **Integrity:** Verify upon receipt of electronically exchanged health information that such information has not been altered and detect the alteration of audit logs.

- **Authentication:** Verify that a person or entity seeking access to electronic health information is the one claimed and is authorized to access such information.

- **Encryption:** Encrypt and decrypt electronic health information in accordance with standards.

- **Accounting of disclosures:** Record disclosures made for treatment, payment, and health care operations (Optional criteria).

Performing a security risk analysis for Meaningful Use

Year 1 criteria to meet Meaningful Use in 2011 or 2012 only contains one privacy and security measure: Conduct or review a security risk analysis per 45 CFR 164.308(a)(1) and implement security updates as necessary.

CFR — Code of Federal Regulations — relates to the requirement in HIPAA to conduct ongoing risk analyses. This means that your security risk analysis should not be something you do only once. Performing a security assessment should be a regular activity. Also, in future years, the security criteria for Meaningful Use will be more stringent.

There isn't any specific guidance provided on what a security risk analysis should entail. This is good in that there isn't an overly burdensome process, but it's also a challenge because there isn't much in terms of specific guidance. Work in partnership with your vendor, Regional Extension Center, or local health system to conduct the security risk analysis, as they have tools, templates, and resources to assist you in conducting the assessment.

Don't despair if your security risk analysis identifies areas that you need to address or remedy. Some common gaps in practices are lack of documented policies and procedures, upgrades to security or virus software, improving the strength of passwords, and ensuring that each user has a unique account.

Getting everyone on board

Your practice's organizational attitude about security should be a part of the overall culture. Here's a couple ways you can get everyone on board with EHR security:

- ✓ **Start with physicians and management personnel.** If they see the importance of meeting privacy and security requirements, they are more apt to champion those measures with office staff, nurses, and medical assistants.

- ✓ **Get employees invested from day one by explaining the importance of the security features and following the EHR-related privacy mandates.** Explain how doing so benefits them and the practice. One way to do this is by including conversations about privacy and security in your initial discussions for EHR adoption.

When you assess your EHR readiness (see Chapter 4), ask questions about how you comply with HIPAA and HITECH regulations and how you can better meet those requirements with an EHR. Ask yourself how you want the EHR to help you meet your privacy and security goals, and make those answers part of the mix when you're reviewing potential vendors.

Asking the right questions

You want to make absolutely sure that your EHR is set up to be as secure and confidential as possible. Make sure that you cover these areas:

✔ **Data and information security**

- Internet technologies are consistent with the latest industry approaches for encryption and authentication

✔ **System support login capabilities**

- Each user in the practice uses his or her own login account (no sharing of user accounts).

- Smart card, proximity card, or token device

- Other security controls and devices, including biometric options such as fingerprints or retinal scans

- Secure remote access methods (Citrix, dialup, Internet) and extent of functionality (complete, view only)

✔ **System functionality**

- Can the system accommodate multiple users on a common workstation with easy login/logout capabilities?

- Can the system log off users automatically after a certain amount of inactivity on a device? How is this function managed?

✔ **System password capabilities**

- Does the user have to change his or her password at set intervals?

- Can IT staff set intervals for password changes to an organization's specifications?

- Are the passwords for the EHR strong passwords — combination of uppercase and lowercase letters, numbers, special characters?

✔ **Role-based access**

- Can the system be configured to limit user access to patient records and functionality based on their role in the organization? For example, can access to patient financial, billing, and medical records information be restricted to only clinical or administrative staff that need to know the information?

- Can certain information, such as psychiatric notes, be hidden from all "inappropriate" users?

- Is there a list of users (or user roles) that can access health information in case of an emergency?

✔ **Monitoring**

- Does the system log all activity to provide a complete audit trail of the specific user, patient, accessed function, date/time, and data change?

- Are record accesses and edits easily reportable by patient and employee?

- Does the application date/time mark entry of all information to show who accessed specific sections of the patient record?

✔ **Network and hardware security**

- Are firewalls or virtual private networks (VPNs) set up or needed?

- Is the wireless network configured to require strong passwords?

- Is the SSID (Service Set Identifier — the secret key to access the network) of the wireless network being broadcasted or is appropriately hidden?

- Is virus protection software installed and up to date on all computers? Is it kept up to date on a regular basis or automatically?

- Are system backups and restores tested on a regular basis?

Your vendor can be one of your closest allies in EHR security. By setting up the most secure EHR controls, you help ensure the protection of your patients' data. And, don't forget, doing so also covers your practice's long-term security costs. When you exercise due diligence to avoid security breaches, you also protect your practice from unwanted penalties and lawsuits.

Securing your perimeter

Here are some specific EHR features that can help you meet your security requirements:

✔ Access restrictions based on categories you can set up and define

✔ Special status indicators for sensitive cases (see the nearby "Handle with care: Who needs extra EHR security?" sidebar for more information)

✔ Ability to assign aliases for sensitive cases

✔ Blocked access for specific notes or reports

✔ Advanced security, tracking, and encryption features for anything accessed remotely (from the physician's home computer, for example)

✔ Encryption and tracking for fax transmissions

✔ Patient record database that can be blocked in the event of a system support event

✔ Troubleshooting that can be activated through use of test data as opposed to live records

✔ Remote support encryption measures

✔ Audit trails that monitor vendor staff activity as well as in-house employee access

✔ Ability to block printing and download of patient data

✔ Multiple levels of data accessibility

✔ Ability to override access restrictions in cases of extreme emergency

Features will differ based on your choice of vendor, but if you see something here you like that your vendor doesn't offer, make a point to let them know. They might add some of those features on the next system update!

Retrofitting old equipment

Many security breaches don't happen as a result of a hacker actively scouting out your new EHR system. Typically, information stored on your old hardware or software gets into the wrong hands by accident. Although you may be excited about fitting your new EHR system with top-of-the-line security features, don't forget about the old PCs from the early '90s, the box of antiquated disk, or the backup drives sitting in the supply closet. If they haven't been properly cleaned of patient records, the sensitive information is there for the taking. Additionally, if you plan to sell old hardware to make room (and earn extra cash) for newer equipment and old files are present on those machines, you're (uh-oh!) in breach of HIPAA regulations and subject to penalties.

These kinds of security breaches, no matter how unintentional, can wreak havoc on your practice and, some say, negate the potential savings of migrating to EHR because of the penalties you'll occur. Therefore, we implore you, take care of your retired hardware. Even old fax machines can retain sensitive information, so nothing is 100 percent clean of data until an IT representative says it is. Find the money to hire a professional who can assure your old equipment is as clean as a newly washed window. You will be glad you did.

Have your IT pro provide you with a Certificate of Data Sanitization so you can prove you did your part to rid old equipment of sensitive data. This is one audit trail you want to keep.

Having a plan going forward

Not one fancy (and secure) bell or whistle will matter if you don't have a plan for addressing future security needs and HIPAA requirements changes. Many of your EHR's security and privacy features are automatic, but that doesn't mean they're entirely intuitive.

You have the technology and processes covered, but don't forget the people who will use those security features. Provide staff ongoing training on privacy rules, legislation, and any security features you add to the EHR. Couple that with your plans to update and upgrade EHR security features to meet HIPAA and HITECH standards, and you have a winning formula for securing your patients' PHI.

Handle with care: Who needs extra EHR security?

Some highly sensitive data warrants enhanced security measures, so keep these categories in mind while you work with your vendor rep to set up your new EHR security features and train your staff:

✔ **Patient Type and Identity:** Your system must be able to authenticate (from inside and outside your office) patient identity and link the patient to the correct records. The PHI record of Mary Jones from Champaign, IL will be very different than Mary Jones from Urbana, IL, so your system must include unique benchmarks that identify both.

✔ **Diagnosis or Condition:** Your system should offer safeguards for especially sensitive diagnoses or conditions. Some examples include mental health, sexually transmitted disease, substance abuse, or chemical dependency.

✔ **Procedure and Testing:** Clinical documentation for controversial procedures, surgeries, family planning (abortions, genetic testing), or cosmetic surgery is especially sensitive.

✔ **Consent and Custody:** The records of patients who cannot consent to disclosures because of health or legal status can benefit from extra security measures. Examples include minors, wards of the state, inmates, incapacitated or incompetent patients, records for the deceased, or parties involved in an adoption.

✔ **Research:** Security features should be implemented for any data created, collected, or reported in support of clinical trials or research.

✔ **Friends, Colleagues, and VIPs:** Many EHRs offer the ability to flag records of VIPs, staff members, or friends of staff. Opening the patient record for a patient flagged as a VIP usually generates an alert notification indicating or inquiring whether the user is authorized to view the patient's record. You've heard the stories of unauthorized access — it's helpful to put safeguards in place to prevent the temptation for your staff and colleagues to look at records they shouldn't be looking at.

According to the Ponemon Institute, a group that conducts independent research on privacy, data protection, and information security policy, investing in a data security plan can create a 432 percent ROI through cost savings alone.

Chapter 11

Training for Success

*T*raining and effective EHR use is a marathon, not a sprint. You might believe that training comprises only the few hours of exposure to the EHR right before you turn it on. However, the training process begins well before you go live and actually continues as long as you use your system. And with each new experience, you build your skills and become more proficient and efficient with the system.

Training sets the foundation for the successful use of the system for you and your practice. Additionally, training events set the tone for overall practice and individual clinician engagement in the EHR process.

Vendors have a significant amount of experience with training practices and offer you a variety of strategies, tools, and methods, including e-learning tools, webinars, and traditional classes to help you implement their EHR successfully. Partner with them to tailor their offerings to meet your specific needs.

Understanding Your Training Needs

Before you start the training, determine what you and your practice specifically require to be successful. Work with your vendor to determine exactly what your practice needs. Ideally, the vendor has previously implemented its product in a practice similar to yours (based on size and specialty) and can identify critical success factors (and obstacles to avoid!).

Keep potential training needs in mind before you make your final vendor selection. Though you may not necessarily know the particulars of what kind of training you want during the vendor selection phase, you can at least ask general questions about what kind of training each vendor offers, what (if any) additional costs are involved, and whether the vendor offers continuing education. See Chapter 6 for information about the vendor selection process.

Here's how to assess your training needs and get the most from the training experience.

✔ **Be an active participant in the training process. Work with the vendor on the following:**

- Training strategies: Discuss pros and cons.

- Are you considering a train-the-trainer approach? Who in your practice are best-suited to be trainers?

- Determining specific functions you and your staff hope to cover in the training.

- Confirming costs for additional training as well as opportunities for continuing education.

✔ **Perform a readiness assessment of your staff and research other data to capture the details of your practice:**

- Are your physicians comfortable with technology or do they think that a mouse is just a rodent that needs to be caught?

- What form of training works best for each stakeholder?

- How does each staff member learn best? Are your colleagues visual, audible, or kinesthetic learners?

- How can you accurately represent all job functions affected by the EHR?

✔ **Gather information important to logistics, such as:**

- Number of staff at each role (physicians, nurse practitioners, RNs, medical assistants, and front desk staff)

- Staff members who don't work full-time at the clinic

- Training space

- Computers for training; you'll need one for each user

- Connectivity for the training room so you can access the electronic training environment

A successful EHR implementation depends on you and your vendor meeting certain responsibilities related to training. Insist the vendor accommodates your needs to enable your success.

Assessing who needs what training

If you are implementing both the clinical electronic health record as well as a new, integrated practice management system, then everyone in your office needs training on the new systems. Even if you're only installing the EHR, most, if not all, of your staff will need some training and access to the EHR, even your front and back office staff. The trick is determining how much training is necessary for each role in your practice.

Consult the workflows that you updated with new procedures and responsibilities. Be sure to include in your training any staff members affected by the implementation. Chapter 8 includes a more detailed review of workflow analysis.

Follow these simple steps to create a chart to plan training for those who need it:

1. **Obtain a list of all training options and classes from the vendor.**
2. **List all roles in your practice.**
3. **Work with the vendor to determine which classes are required and which ones are only suggested.**
4. **Communicate the training options to your staff along with expectations for their attendance.**

   Consider making a chart, similar to the one shown in Figure 11-1, so everyone knows what training is expected of them.

		Physician	Nurse	Office Manager	Medical Assistant	Front Office
eLearning	EMR Basics	R	R	R	R	
	ePrescribing	S	S	S		
	Decision Support	S	S	S		
	Front Office			S		S
	Patient Documents		S	S		S
	Scheduling			S		
Webinars	Specialty Forms		S	S	S	
	Referral Management	S	S	S		S
	ePrescribing	S		S		
	Check In			S	S	S
	Check Out			S		S
	Advanced Ordering	S		S		
Class Training	Front Office			R		R
	EMR Basics	R	R	R	R	
	EMR Intermediate	R	R	R		

S = Suggested   R = Required

Figure 11-1: Determining training needs for your staff.

Confirming your trainers

In most implementations, the vendor performs the majority of the training because they have the experience and resources. However, if your practice is very large or you're part of a multipractice installation, the vendor might bring in additional training help from an outside source. If that's the case, be sure to confirm who your trainers will be and what their qualifications are before you get in a classroom with them.

Trainers who've worked in an office, especially clinicians, generally provide greater value to you and your practice. They have a significant advantage over other trainers because they understand office workflows, can anticipate potential issues, and respond knowledgeably to most questions.

You should also identify a super user from your staff who can take over future training for new staff or provide follow-up training for all end users. A super user is a member of your staff who is particularly adept at using the practice's EHR system and can teach others to use the technology. Read more about super users and how to identify them in the upcoming "Developing your own talent" section.

Develop a super user for each role so that each super user can focus on supporting his or her peers: physician, nurse, medical assistant, front office, back office. Depending upon the size of your practice, you may consider more than one super user per role to cover for any staff turnover. After all, if you only have one, and that person leaves your practice, you may incur additional training costs to train a new super user.

Incorporating workflows and functionality into training

Training is about much more than just learning to click a button or tab, or navigate to a section in your EHR. Valuable training addresses how you and your practice deliver care and how that care delivery process is affected by the new EHR. Usually, most questions after you turn on the system relate to workflow and processes, not system functionality.

The vendor doesn't know your specific office processes; they need your help to identify, modify, and incorporate your workflows into training. Someone from your staff should participate in each of the training classes, take on the responsibility of answering workflow questions, and help the vendor teach those workflows.

Most, if not all, vendor systems allow you to accomplish the same task several ways. Make decisions for the practice about which way to train. If you train multiple ways, the training will likely confuse your colleagues and staff rather than help prepare them to use the EHR.

Understanding the Vendor's Role in Training

Luckily, the responsibility of training doesn't solely rest on your shoulders. The vendor can and should be an active participant in the process, leading the way and offering a wide variety of training options that best serve your staff's needs. You negotiated training as part of the vendor selection and contract negotiations (Chapters 6 and 7, respectively). Check your contract for the vendor's training role and responsibilities, including

- ✔ **Hours:** Number of training hours, including a breakdown of hours by staff member role
- ✔ **Personnel:** Number of facilitators, including background and experience level
- ✔ **Methods:** Classes, e-learning modules, webinars, and so on
- ✔ **Location:** Remote or in person
- ✔ **Timing:** Phased training is always recommended — some training should occur before go-live (during implementation, before preloading), additional training should occur just prior to go-live, and supplemental/ re-training should occur a few months after go-live
- ✔ **Responsibility for developing materials:** Who develops classroom training manuals, practice scenarios, tip sheets, e-learning, and so on

A vendor should meet you more than halfway and offer the training scenarios that you want to implement. Request reports from each test initiative to review and chart everyone's progress and pinpoint areas of concern. Find out how your vendor training program charts attendance and training performance and request these reports frequently. The vendor's success depends on your successful transition to EHR so he should comply with all your requests.

Knowing what the vendor can do

Vendors are a tremendous resource and help your practice in many ways, but they can't do everything training-related for you. Understand their strengths and their limitations and keep your expectations of their role reasonable. Ask them to provide material specific to you. Don't be afraid to ask the vendor to tailor their training material to suit your specific practice and specialty.

Ask the vendor to

- Present training options; include pros and cons and any additional costs
- Provide a training strategy and timeline
- Set up a training environment with test patients and appropriate practice scenarios
- Provide example proficiency testing options and recommendations
- Communicate any specific requirements for training; for example, room reservations, food, projector, flip charts, and other helpful technology or materials
- Coordinate training sessions with the practice manager or clinical lead
- Provide references for their overall training and for the specific trainers they propose assist your practice.

Interviewing the vendor team

In the course of selecting your vendor, you conducted interviews with their leadership, the project teams, and their references. Continue exercising due diligence with the resource people whom they propose train you and your staff.

Ask the following questions of the potential trainers:

- How long have you been a trainer?
- How long have you been training these specific modules/applications?
- Describe the process that you went through to become a trainer.
- Do you have a clinical or office practice background? If so, please elaborate.
- How have you handled a disgruntled training attendee?
- What makes you a good trainer?

Conduct reference checks with practices that have been live for a few months. Ask the following questions of a reference:

- What was your experience with your trainer?
- What did they do well?
- What do you wish they would have done differently?
- Were there any specific problems with any training class attendees? If so, how did they handle the situation?
- Would you request them again to train your staff?

Reviewing the training materials

Only you know your practice and how you and your staff deliver care. Make sure that the training materials reflect that and ensure that your workflows are embedded in the training. All the materials, including the main training manual, e-learning modules, pocket guides, and exercises, are key components of the complete training. Each training element is best utilized during different stages of your implementation and serves a distinct purpose.

Table 11-1 describes the types of training materials and characteristics to look for during your evaluation and review process.

Table 11-1	Training Materials	
Material	*Description*	*What to Look For*
Training manual	Most-detailed materials reviewing all EHR system functionality; ideally tailored to your specialty, practice, and specific workflows; for use with instructor in classroom and remote training sessions	The material is relevant both clinically and to your practice; practice-specific workflows are embedded; the materials are easy to follow; the materials contain screenshots with step-by-step descriptions
E-learning modules	Focused on specific functionality or workflows; may not be specific to your specialty or even version of the software; great for initial exposure to the system or for use to review specific EHR tools; available remotely and can be accessed at any time	The materials are easily assessable; the modules are appropriate in length and content (most useful modules range between 5 and 20 minutes); the modules are interactive and allow the end user to participate in the sessions
Quick reference guides (trifolds/ pocket guides)	Step-by-step guides for key workflows or system functions; specific to your practice and specialty; used most during the go-live period and immediately thereafter; not meant to cover all EHR functions or clinical workflows	The major EHR functions are covered; the guide is brief with easy to follow steps; the guides are portable

(continued)

Table 11-1 (continued)

Material	Description	What to Look For
Exercises	Specific tools for end users to review and practice their new EHR skills; focus on clinically relevant work-flows; reinforce key system features and functions; for use as part of the classroom training and practice sessions prior to go-live	The exercises are clinically accurate and specific to your patient population; they cover all key system features

If you can, have one representative from each role (RN, front desk staff, and physician) review the materials and participate in the first training class. Super users are a good choice here. Make sure that there is enough time between that first class and the remainder of the training so that the vendor can incorporate your feedback into future training.

Understanding Methods and Methodologies

Vendors utilize many strategies and methods to accomplish training. With their help, tailor their offerings to meet the needs and specific requirements of your practice.

Forming training classes

You can group your staff in multiple ways to get the most out of training:

✔ **Role based:** Structure classes by job role (RN, front desk staff, and physician). The trainer focuses on the specific workflows for each role and allows the attendees to ask appropriate questions. A downside to role-based training is that end users may not focus on or be trained in the multidisciplinary workflows or understand how each person contributes to the documentation of the office visit.

✔ **Team:** Group attendees in a class with their team of physician, nurse, and medical assistant. Each attendee is trained on the entire workflow and how each staff member contributes to the EHR. Some of the questions and workflows are not going to be relevant to all end users, but it can be useful for everyone to see how their workflows are interrelated.

✔ **Specialty:** Focus on workflows, content, and questions that relate only to a specialty, such as internal medicine, cardiology, or general surgery. Training is similar to role-based training, but allows the end users to obtain a deeper understanding of the content and workflows.

Many practices successfully combine role-based training and team training to provide a robust, complete training experience. For example, if you have eight hours of training, conduct six hours in role-based training and two hours in team training.

Provide a separate one-on-one training session for physicians who might not be as facile with a computer as others in your practice. No one likes to appear inept, especially physicians who've spent their entire lives excelling.

Picking the right training options

The vendors provide a variety of training options for practices and you can pick one method, or more likely a combination of classes, that fit your specific needs. Check out the EHR training menu:

✔ **In-person classes:** Classes provide the most robust training for you and your staff. A trainer meets with your staff and walks you through the training materials while you follow along on a computer. You decide who attends the classes — a clinical team of nurses, all medical assistants and physicians, a group of physicians, or maybe just one physician at a time. The downside is that these classes are usually the most expensive option, but you'll have direct access to the trainer to ask follow-up and specific questions.

✔ **Remote classes:** Designed in a similar fashion as the in-person classes, but the trainer leads a class from an offsite location using Web-conferencing tools. Remote classes are cheaper than onsite training that's done in person. If you have well-trained super users, it may be a good idea to have a few remote classes for follow-up training (post go-live) or for new clinicians or staff.

✔ **E-learning modules:** Modules are for individual use and accessed when it's convenient for the end user. Most vendors have their own modules, and some practices develop their own. You can use these modules to serve a variety of purposes; most of all, e-learning serves as a good approach for supplemental learning:

  • Teach basic information about the EHR prior to training

  • Keep end users proficient before they go-live but after their training

  • Refresh end users on specific topics after they go-live

✔ **Webinars:** These are topic-specific, live Internet sessions where you can ask questions of the instructor; however, the sessions may not cover the exact same software version you choose and may include participants from all over the country. If you want something tailored to your staff, the in-person or remote class setups might be a better option. Figure 11-2 shows what a webinar looks like.

✔ **Computer training:** Not everyone is experienced in working with a computer — you may need to have some basic computer skills training for your team. Determine whether this is something that can be done by someone in your practice or whether you need to employ the skills of an experienced trainer either in a classroom setting or onsite. Assess computer proficiency early during the planning process so you can budget costs and time to bring people with limited familiarity with computers up to speed.

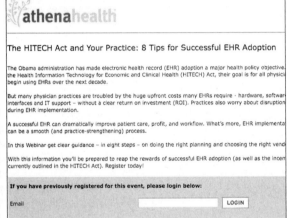

Figure 11-2: A webinar offered by a vendor for education purposes.

Give everyone time to complete their e-learning and webinar sessions. Provide schedule relief for all staff members to encourage their participation.

Completing the Training

You've planned appropriately and made all the necessary decisions. You've assessed the readiness of your staff and determined the appropriate class size and participants. Your materials are clinically relevant and easy to understand. You and your staff are enthusiastic — well, maybe not enthusiastic, but at least willing to complete the training.

A few ground rules for a successful training session:

> ✔ **Schedule the time in advance and clear everyone's schedule.** For many offices, this means closing for a half day or coming in on a Saturday to complete the training. You need everyone's undivided attention and don't want any distractions to take away from the training.
>
> ✔ **Provide food.** It may sound silly, but food is an easy way to entice participation for the event. Chocolate doesn't hurt, either. Lots of chocolate.
>
> ✔ **Respect and value the participants' time.**
>
> > • Start and end the training on time.
> >
> > • Follow a detailed agenda.
> >
> > • Capture issues and questions and follow up appropriately and have them on hand during go-live.
> >
> > • Manage the expectations of your staff and don't let the vendor mismanage those expectations by making any promises they can't deliver.
>
> ✔ **Incorporate feedback from earlier sessions.** If you're providing more than one training session, listen to your staff and colleagues and implement their changes and requests before subsequent classes commence.
>
> Develop an FAQ based upon questions and issues from prior training sessions or practice experiences.

Deciding when to train

When's the right time to provide training? Do you train four to six weeks ahead of your go-live or wait until one to two days before you turn on the system? Although both strategies can work, most practices (and individuals) do much better if training is closer to go-live so the information is fresh in everyone's mind. (Some preliminary work will have to be done in regard to preloading and scanning charts, too, which you read about in Chapter 9.) Ask the vendor to accommodate your requests for training near go-live or provide rationale for the alternative strategy.

Scheduling training time

Total training time is based on a few factors, including amount of functionality that you are implementing, EHR experience of your staff, and complexity of the EHR. Neither you nor your staff will retain everything you learn, and you shouldn't be expected to. Build a foundation, learn the basic skills, and make a commitment to improve with time.

Depending on the amount of training that is necessary for you and your staff, the vendor may offer to split the training into multiple sessions or complete it all in one sitting. If you get the choice, and the training is for more than four hours, split the classes into two or three days. After four hours, your retention of the material decreases significantly. Additionally, at the subsequent classes, you can start with a refresher of the previous class to reinforce your skills and knowledge.

Complete an assessment of your staff prior to training and group training class attendees by their computer skills and previous EHR experience. If all the "expert" users are in a class together, the trainer may be able to accelerate the class.

Implementing the seeing, doing, and doing again process

With some minor modifications, the adage "See one, do one, teach one" from your medical education also applies to your EHR training. You can help ensure you and your staff knows how to use the system when you follow those steps during training:

1. **See one:** Watch the trainer go through a clinical scenario and do not try to follow along on your computer. Focus on the trainer.

   An example might be placing an order for labs and medications for your test patient.

2. **Do one with the trainer:** Go through the same example with the trainer using different labs and medications.

   The trainer can walk through the scenario while you follow along on your computer.

3. **Do one on your own:** Execute the same steps on your own until you feel comfortable with the technology.

Use appropriate clinical scenarios during the training. If you can connect your learning to a clinical example, you're significantly more likely to retain that knowledge.

Testing proficiency

Test how well each staff member can use the EHR and absorb the training materials. Don't expect everyone to be an expert but do confirm that everyone has the basic skills to care for patients using this new system. Measuring the proficiency of your staff serves several purposes:

✔ Identifies users who need additional training or support.

✔ Identifies specific areas of training that may be unclear. If users are consistently missing questions in one area, the curriculum or the proficiency test needs to be evaluated and potentially adjusted.

✔ Provides an official measurement of the success of training.

Conduct the proficiency test at the end of the training class. If someone doesn't pass the test, identify whether additional education in a specific area is needed or whether a global concern might warrant a review with all participants or additional guidance from the vendor.

Staying proficient before go-live

If training occurs weeks before go-live, forgetting everything you learned during training is easy. Fortunately, you can employ a number of strategies to keep you and your practice proficient.

In Chapter 9, we discuss strategies for preloading pertinent patient information into the EHR prior to go-live. In addition to creating the foundation of the clinical record for many of your patients, this preload process offers a great opportunity for staff to play in the system and become more comfortable.

Don't use a form or method of entering information from the paper chart that doesn't mimic the workflow that staff and physicians will use after you turn on the EHR. You want to reinforce the workflows from your training and help build upon your strong foundation.

You can also practice in the system to keep your skills sharp. Make the practice effective by working with test patients who have robust data; use clinically accurate practice scenarios, too. Ask the vendor to provide practice documents for your review and tweak them as appropriate to fit your practice.

Schedule the time for staff and physicians to go through e-learning modules or practice scenarios. Make it clear that the "free" time is for practice and not other clinical or non-clinical tasks. If the physicians are paid based on productivity or Relative Value Units (RVUs), then provide relief or compensation. The return you get on the time investment is well worth the cost.

Continuing to Learn on the Job

The pre–go-live training and the go-live itself are just the beginning of the EHR learning process, and obtaining both clinical and financial value requires constant learning. When you first start using the EHR, you don't have to use all the tricks and advanced functionality of the system. You need to get through your days, keep your patients healthy, and maintain your sanity. And then, little by little, you can get better and more proficient at using the EHR to document care delivery and manage your patients.

Create a strategy for ongoing training and education with your vendor and establish clear responsibilities and expectations for them. Determine timing, resources, and scope of future formalized training, and communicate that throughout your practice. You can also supplement the extra classroom training with specific e-learning modules and webinars.

Developing your own talent

Even the best and most responsive vendor can't and shouldn't do everything for you. Your long-term success depends on cultivating your own group of the following experts who can support your end users and lead your optimization efforts:

- ✔ **Super users:** A super user is particularly adept at using the practice's EHR system and can teach others to use the technology. Additionally, they can serve as "champions" of the system and act as built-in technical support for other members of your staff. The super user should have extensive knowledge of the software and the workflows of the departments in the office. The number of super users you need depends on the size of your practice. With a large practice, you may need to train a super user in each staff role; with a small practice, you may need to train only one or two staff members.

  After you identify the staff member(s) with the appropriate combination of technical savvy and willingness and ability to teach, you must ensure they're provided with adequate training. Because they will be asked to perform far beyond their peers, they'll require education that's much more extensive than what's given to their colleagues.

  During go-live, relieve the super user of other practice duties in order to focus specifically on technical support. At go-live, the super users serve as the first line of response to staff with issues or questions.

- ✔ **Trainer:** Many vendors employ a strategy of "train the trainer" to help practices build their internal team and appropriately offload some of the long-term training responsibility to the practice. Programs vary by vendor, but may include classes at the vendor site for two to four weeks. These intensive courses provide a robust learning environment for your trainers and allow you to build the internal team to support your practice with limited vendor support.

Invest in building your own team. The long-term cost is lower, you and your staff will be more proficient users, and you obtain more value from your EHR.

Everyone is always busy, but it's important to stress that training is mandatory for your practice. You do not want to go-live with clinicians or staff who have not completed adequate training — it will negatively affect productivity, the untrained individual will be frustrated or require increased support, and it may cast an overall negative impression about the EHR. Withhold users from getting logon credentials until after the requisite amount of training; they can't practice or work until they've completed training. Determine what the best way is to motivate your practice to be adequately trained — it will make a successful EHR adoption.

Training post–go-live

When new members join your staff, they must be properly trained on how to use your system. Identify a staff member responsible for that training, how long the training will last, and what training method you will use.

A super user is an ideal person to perform the training. Arrange coverage or schedule the new-hire's training time after regular business hours so training time doesn't conflict with the super user's normal work.

Staff will likely develop tips, tricks, and shortcuts to share with colleagues. Additionally, the vendor will continuously upgrade the software, mostly based on feedback from individual practices. Stay abreast of changes, have someone in the practice responsible for ensuring this information is properly disseminated, and offer formal training when appropriate.

You'll have to put together an ongoing training strategy to train employees on new features as your system gets upgraded. Your super user is an ideal candidate to lead this training, as well.

The learning never ends, and that's actually a good thing for most clinicians. The systems will continually evolve; you have the opportunity to grow with them and improve your ability to deliver quality patient care.

Chapter 12

Communicating and Marketing Your EHR

*A*n important part of your EHR adoption and implementation process is communicating the news that your practice has joined the electronic revolution. Doing so provides a terrific opportunity to connect with patients and the public about your new EHR and your organization. Your initial EHR-related communications can set the tone for your overall communication strategy going forward.

Harris Interactive reports that a mere 16 percent of U.S. adults have discussed an EHR with their healthcare provider. Who knows why that number is so low, but one thing is for certain — communicating changes your practice is going through to patients and getting them on board with all things electronic can be a challenge. But it's one that you must address if you want patients to buy into the new EHR reality. You want patients to become comfortable with the idea of having their health records exist in e-form. You also want them to understand that by using an EHR, they can more actively participate in their healthcare management. Your goal is to allay their concerns about privacy and security and get them invested in the benefits EHR has to offer them.

Your patients have the potential to be some of your biggest EHR champions outside the office. Approach the EHR issue with them in a positive way that allows them to participate in their own care.

Knowing What to Tell Patients about Your New EHR

You and your staff have been positively bombarded with EHR information over the last few months, and chances are good you're suffering from information overload. You may be tempted to share your new wealth of EHR information with everyone you meet — you're practically an expert, after all. But please save the massive info download for your dog, cat, or bird. When relaying information about your practice's new system to patients, keep the communication simple, straightforward, and directed to the patients' concerns and interests. Ideally, you should touch on four areas with your patients:

- ✔ What, exactly, the EHR is and does
- ✔ Privacy and security concerns
- ✔ How the EHR benefits patients
- ✔ What role the patient can play with the EHR

Harris Interactive and Xerox Corporation conducted a survey in which almost half of the 2,180 people polled said EHRs would make healthcare delivery more efficient but didn't know how EHR would affect them as patients.

Defining EHR for your patients

An EHR's purpose and function may seem obvious to you, but to most people, EHR is a foreign term. Until patients enter your practice, they probably don't think much about electronic health records, what they are, and what they actually do.

Provide a simple, easy-to-understand explanation of what the system is and what it does. Keep your EHR definition simple and, regardless of how you want to impart the information, tell your patients the following:

- ✔ EHR stands for electronic health records.
- ✔ An EHR is all your health records saved in electronic form.
- ✔ You no longer have a paper chart.
- ✔ Important information from your paper chart will transfer to the EHR.
- ✔ EHRs are private, safe, and secure.
- ✔ Your health can benefit from the EHR.

To help your patients familiarize themselves with the EHR and become comfortable with the idea of electronically housing their PHI (personal health information), communicate to them what the EHR does. Include these EHR features and functions in your explanation:

- ✔ EHRs contain decision support logic to check for allergies and medication interactions.

- ✔ EHRs allow viewing and graphing of patient data over time, making understanding patient progress and health easier.

- ✔ EHR accepts scans of important patient information, such as insurance cards, reports, and test results and then imports them into the EHR.

- ✔ EHRs can print all kinds of helpful materials, such as a summary of patient visits or a list of recommended services (like shots or screenings).

- ✔ EHRs allow communication of information to outside health professionals (like specialists or pharmacists) to provide care.

- ✔ All patient prescriptions and refill orders can be managed online and transmitted to the pharmacy by using an EHR.

- ✔ EHRs use features like secure messaging (similar to e-mail) or automated phone messaging to communicate important information to patients (such as appointment reminders).

- ✔ Billing and insurance claims use the EHR to achieve better accuracy.

- ✔ Physicians can use the EHR to set up specialist referrals.

Don't relay every single bell and whistle to your patients. Hit the highlights and explain the EHR system's capabilities in simple, straightforward terms.

Addressing privacy concerns

The security and privacy of PHI will likely be a concern for patients. Reassure patients that their information is secure and accessible only by the healthcare professionals who need to access it — which was the case with their paper records.

Focus on the positive aspects of provider accessibility when you remind patients that their information is secure. The EHR helps promote faster coordination between providers (regardless of physical location), more efficient care, and gives patients access to their own information.

Who has access to their information, how it can be accessed, and what level of control they have over their PHI will be at the top of everyone's "to ask" list. Be ready for those questions and, more importantly, be proactive about disseminating information about your security plan to your patients. Write a security FAQ, create a brochure, hold a Q&A session (both in person and via podcast), post flyers, and simply answer questions during office visits in order to fill your clients in.

According to a Harris Interactive 2010 survey, 79 percent of adults who have concerns about digital medical records report stolen records as their number one concern, followed by misuse of information (69 percent), and lost or damaged records (68 percent).

Discuss with patients the following information about EHR security and privacy:

- ✔ EHRs can only be viewed by approved staff with security access codes.

- ✔ EHRs have many types of security settings. Only certain people can see all your health information. Office staff might only see such information as your name and contact information, for example.

- ✔ Patients sign a consent form that details who can view their PHI.

- ✔ If there is ever a concern, you can always run a report to see exactly who accessed a patient's chart and when.

- ✔ Physicians can enter private notes in a patient record that only the physician can read.

You don't have to share everything you know about EHR privacy and security with the patient. An overview, including how the EHR security features work, will be sufficient.

Survey says . . .

A recent survey conducted by Harris Interactive and HealthDay reports that 78 percent of U.S. adults "strongly agree" or "somewhat agree" that physicians should have access to their electronic medical records, and 71 percent could envision themselves using the EHR to manage their own health. Of those surveyed, though, only 28 percent said their primary care physician used electronic records. Forty-two percent said they have a primary care physician, but were unsure whether he or she used electronic records.

While most consumers (patients) have a basic understanding of what an EHR is and does, the majority do not understand how an EHR can benefit them personally. You, the practice's EHR champion, can bridge the awareness gap for patients by creating your own grassroots marketing campaign to help them harness the power of electronic records.

Explaining the benefits

To get your patients on board the EHR bandwagon, explain the benefits the EHR offers them, too. Yes, many of the benefits are for the practice, but patients can get a lot from the system, too, if they're open to the new experience of managing their care in an electronic environment. By outlining the EHR's benefits to your patience, you leverage their privacy and security concerns and gain valuable trust.

You're not in this alone. Check with your REC for help with setting up your practice's patient outreach program or get tips from other practices or hospitals that have already gone live.

Your primary message to patients should be that they can use the EHR to participate in their own care. Immediate access to patient records allows physicians to display information on the spot to answer questions, confirm information accuracy, and brainstorm ideas with the patient. You should relay that information, among other beneficial activities, to your patients. No matter what kind of communication campaign you use, the message should be the same across the board: Your patients receive short-term and long-term benefits from using the EHR. Here are some common benefits to highlight for your patients:

- ✔ Faster and more efficient office visits.

- ✔ Better accuracy in chart notes; fewer handwriting issues that cause errors.

- ✔ Quicker availability of labs and test results.

- ✔ Physicians can instantly share test results with outside specialists, creating better communication that results in better quality of care.

- ✔ Patients can access their medical records, including lab results and immunization history, online.

- ✔ Access for approved parties to healthcare records. For example, parents can access a child's health records (such as immunizations) online. This is especially useful when parents have to print or send records for school, daycare, and sports programs. Or people managing their parents' care can access their healthcare records.

- ✔ Medication list can generate drug reaction and interaction issues.

- ✔ Streamlined prescription processes make it faster and easier to pick up prescriptions and order refills.

- ✔ Save money on prescriptions by reviewing medication lists and costs with the physician.

- ✔ E-mail reminders help patients remember upcoming appointments and care concerns.

- ✔ Patients can receive e-mail or phone calls regarding emerging research that affects patient conditions.

Be sure to remind patients that the EHR can be used as a great communication tool during the office visit by allowing the patient a view into their own health record. A physician should maintain strong eye contact with the patient, place the monitor so it is accessible to both, and engage the patient while they view the EHR.

Communicating Appropriately

Pick a medium, any medium. No matter how you choose to communicate information about the new EHR to your patients, the message remains the same — you're committed to providing them a safe, secure, quality healthcare experience. To gain your patients' trust and their buy-in, offer your clients EHR information in a personable way. Use a friendly, conversational manner in verbal communication and printed marketing materials. Remember your job isn't to relay everything you know about the EHR and how it works. Your job (at least right now) is to communicate information about something that can be quite complicated in an easy-to-understand and friendly way.

Run some demographic numbers on your patient population before you create a marketing campaign to present your EHR. You can determine the tone of your overall message based on whom you serve and how comfortable they are with technology before you overwhelm them with EHR educational materials.

Checking the pulse of your communication

You may be so intensely focused on communicating *about* your EHR to your patients that you overlook how you communicate with them *using* the EHR. Your brochures aren't worth much unless you can communicate with your patients during office visits using both verbal and non-verbal skills.

Many physicians are hesitant to use an EHR because they don't want their personal interactions with patients to suffer. According to a 2001 article from the American Medical Informatics Association, physicians who use an EHR were more likely to ask questions and clarify health information but less likely to ask about emotional

or psychosocial issues. They found information-related tasks easier to accomplish, but were less adept at the relationship-related aspects of communication. However, another study showed there was a correlation between more accurate physician explanations of diagnoses and treatments and positive perceptions of patient involvement in healthcare management.

To overcome any EHR-related communications hiccups, you can set clear expectations with office staff on the appropriateness of electronic and oral communication. Remind your staff that the EHR is a cool new toy, but nothing can replace face-to-face, engaged interaction.

You want to keep your EHR-related patient communications simple, conversational, and direct. Try an approach that includes print, Web-based, and verbal communications. This way, you reach multiple audiences and all types of learners.

There are different kinds of learners. Some people respond to auditory messages; others are visual learners. Creating EHR communications in multiple formats is important to reach all your audiences in a way that best helps them process the information.

Creating pamphlets

Creating a pamphlet that helps you communicate information about your new EHR really isn't as scary as it sounds. You can use many programs to create a quick, easy-to-read pamphlet about your new EHR, and many of them are free or included with your computer. Most of them offer preset templates so you can drop your text into an existing design. *Voilà!* Instant pamphlet! Here are some options to check out:

- ✔ **Web-based publishing software and templates:** You can download these free software options from the Internet: Open Office, Scribus, My Brochure Maker, and Brochure Monster.

- ✔ **Word processing programs:** These programs are preloaded on your computer, or you can install from a CD/DVD: Microsoft Word, Microsoft Works, iWork, and WordPerfect. You may find free versions, but you should look into the paid versions to get their full capabilities. Word processing programs aren't meant to create brochures, so you'll most likely go through some trial and error to get the look you want.

- ✔ **Desktop publishing programs:** These programs are dedicated page layout programs that you install from a CD/DVD: Adobe InDesign, PagePlus, The Print Shop, Print Artist, PrintMaster, Microsoft Publisher, Print Workshop, and Design & Print. These are high-end programs that require some expertise to use. But you can create some fancy brochures with these programs.

You can also use an outside resource to help you create a patient information pamphlet if you're strapped for time and resources. If you're not already working with a graphic design firm or print shop for other office needs (such as business cards and letterhead), check with local companies to get quotes and sample brochures.

Regardless of how you choose to create the document, you're responsible for coming up with the content. Focus on your "big three" topics: defining EHR, privacy and security, and patient benefits.

Offer your patient brochure in multiple languages (Spanish, at the very least) in case you have patients who are non-English speakers.

After your pamphlets or brochures are printed, give them to each patient who comes into the practice after go-live. You should also make the pamphlets available at various locations throughout the office, especially in the lobby and in each examination room. Another option for reaching your entire patient population is to enclose a pamphlet with each bill your office sends. This gets the message out more quickly to patients who visit the office infrequently.

Outlining talking points

When talking to your patients, the last thing you want to do is leave your patients with that "deer in the headlights" look because you fit everything you know about EHR into a 15-minute conversation. Craft only some talking points about the new EHR to communicate with patients.

You also don't want to say too little or just hand off your info pamphlet and call it a day. Instead, train office staff and physicians to explain what they're doing with patients during their day-to-day interactions. Instruct them to be ready to answer general questions about the EHR and if they don't know the answer, either direct patients to someone who does or find the answer and report back to the patient. These types of interactions don't have to be full-on tutorials — they can be simple asides or casual chats. Create a FAQ document so that everyone provides the same answers and can refer to the sheet if necessary. Remember to reduce your schedule at go-live so you and your staff have more time to talk with each patient.

Here are some talking points each role can cover with patients during clinical interactions:

- ✔ **Front office staff:** Your front office staff should relay introductory information about the EHR — what EHR means and does. Have them explain their role in using the EHR: scanning forms and insurance cards, setting up appointments, and following up on patient calls. Staff can relay patient benefits, such as faster and more efficient office visits, greater accessibility to medical records, automated appointment reminders, and more accurate and timely billing and coding.

- ✔ **Intake staff:** Your intake staff can show patients the EHR screens and explain or demo the tasks they perform during intake, such as entering vitals, entering patient concerns or questions for the physician, and confirming any existing health issues or history. They can report patient benefits, such as less time waiting during the intake process, viewing patients' vitals history onscreen, and requesting and printing patient education information during the visit.

✔ **Nursing staff:** Nurses can show the patient how they use the EHR to record data, pull up test results, and coordinate with outside entities using the EHR. They can also report patient benefits, such as better accuracy in chart notes, fewer mistakes caused by handwriting errors, and quicker availability of labs and test results.

✔ **Physicians:** Physicians can show patients their charts onscreen, demonstrate how they pull up histories/lab reports/diagnostic imaging, show patients how they can access their own health records offsite and print or request education information. Test results can be instantly shared between the physician and outside specialists, creating better communication that results in better quality of care. They can report patient benefits, such as streamlined prescription processes, ability to actively discuss records with the physician at the time of visit, talk about drug reaction or interaction issues by viewing the medication list, ability to access online educational articles during visits, save money on prescriptions by viewing medication lists and costs with the physician, and view their own records and access other online health information during the visit, which allows for their questions to be answered in person.

You never know what patients might ask you about the EHR, so you can't solely rely on your rehearsed EHR answers to get you through. The following is a sampling of EHR questions you might be asked and should be ready to answer:

✔ How does your e-prescribing system work?

✔ Can I request refills online?

✔ Who, outside of this office, can access my health information?

✔ How do you communicate with outside specialists?

✔ Why do you get government incentives for using an EHR?

✔ Where can I get more information about how EHRs can help me?

✔ What kind of educational materials can you print for me?

✔ What can we view together onscreen?

✔ How does the EHR save me money?

✔ Can I access my child's/parent's health records if I'm their primary caregiver?

Any time you and your staff chat with a patient about your practice's new system is an opportunity to create another EHR champion. This time, though, the champion can leave your office and spread the word to other consumer stakeholders. So impart the information that is most accurate, most direct, and most useful for your patients.

Keeping updates on your Web site

As long as you're making the move to EHR, take the time to establish or update your practice's Web site with all your EHR information.

Your main goals and talking points shouldn't differ greatly from the information you impart in print and in person. Hit the same highlights so you can create a universal message about your EHR.

Create a dedicated page about EHR information on your Web site and linking to it from the home page (see Figure 12-1). Your EHR page can house the FAQ, online demos or podcasts, links to consumer-appropriate webinars, and examples of documents or forms. The FAQ should anticipate some of patients' most pointed questions about the new EHR, including questions about documentation, tasks, results, billing, patient benefits, security, access, and what happens if the system goes down. Figure 12-2 shows a FAQ page.

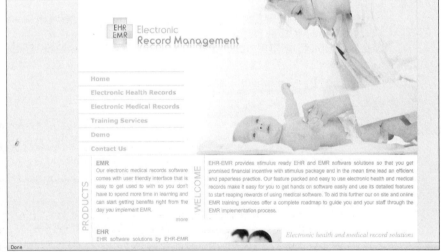

Figure 12-1:
A home page that links to an EHR resource page.

Communication Do's and Don'ts

All this communicating might make you feel like you and your practice are an open book and, in the case of the EHR, that's a good thing! When explaining this new system to patients, you want to be as open as possible and maintain a level of clinical professionalism in which you don't over share — a tough balance. Keep some general do's and don'ts in mind to help you get patients on board with your practice's move to EHR.

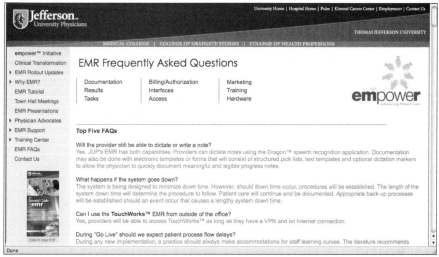

Here are some ways to help your communications strategy achieve its goals:

- ✔ Keep your message positive. Don't complain about the EHR in front of your patients.

- ✔ Make patients feel like they're part of the team.

- ✔ Manage expectations.

- ✔ Define EHR in terms of what it does for the patient.

- ✔ Tell patients how you use electronic features to enhance their patient experience. For example, let them know how, exactly, sending messages electronically is more efficient and safer than sticking a sticky note to their chart.

- ✔ Use demonstrations when appropriate. Explain what you're doing so patients don't feel like you're spending their face time typing. If, for example, you have to add several notations to a record, you can say, "I have to enter your symptoms so that we can diagnose you more accurately."

- ✔ Ask patients whether they have questions or concerns.

- ✔ If patients have more questions, provide the name of a contact person.

- ✔ Follow any EHR explanations with an open-ended question, such as, "What else can I answer for you?" to keep the conversation going.

- ✔ Find the answer to a patient's question if you don't know it already. Follow up.

- ✔ Address individual privacy or security concerns.

- ✔ Explain that, at first, using the EHR may make things go a bit slower.

✔ Anticipate complaints and deal with them objectively on a case-by-case basis.

✔ Offer your patient communication in multiple forms — print, Web, verbal.

✔ Take your patients' EHR temperature after the go-live. Conduct a brief patient survey or simply ask patients about any changes or concerns they've noted since you began using the EHR to manage their care.

To keep your EHR message positive when outlining the details of the new system to your patients, there are some no-no's. Keep the following don'ts in mind when communicating with your patients:

✔ Don't assume patients understand clinical or technical jargon.

✔ Don't expect very sick patients to want to discuss the EHR in detail. They feel terrible and probably don't care at that moment.

✔ Don't make patients feel uncomfortable by oversimplifying your message or ignoring their concerns.

✔ Don't overwhelm patients with technical information. Remember to keep your message directed to what they need to know.

✔ Don't downplay what may seem to be outrageous or offbeat concerns. If Mr. Jones really thinks the FBI is checking up on his health records as part of a vast conspiracy, try to allay his "unique" concerns with sensitivity and compassion.

✔ Don't expect everyone to be enthusiastic about the change. Some people just won't be on board with having their information saved in an electronic environment. Move on.

Everyone processes information differently, so what may be a unique communication concern for one patient may be a non-issue for another. Alter these do's and don'ts on a case-by-case basis, depending on the conversation you're having with each patient and the medium you're using (print, verbal, or Web). The one thread, though, is your "big three" message: definition, privacy and security, and patient benefits. Make it your mantra.

They experience many of the benefits associated with having their records in electronic form. So, it's no wonder that they also have the potential to provide your practice with some true grassroots marketing. It may take some time for you and your patients to be completely comfortable so don't be surprised if they're not shouting from the rooftops after day one.

If your patients express to you that they feel their quality of care has improved or that their visits seem more streamlined with the new EHR, then you have an opportunity to ask them to share that information. You should be able to tell which patients like your new EHR by how they respond when they're in the office, so be aware of those good vibes and make them work for your practice.

Oops! A snapshot of communications gone wrong

You probably believe you're telling patients everything they need or want to know about the migration to EHR and that the new system is working out perfectly for them. Perhaps, as you are asking them how their care has improved since your go-live, they've responded with a rote "Fine." But, what if you're misreading the situation? The results of a survey by Massachusetts Health Quality Partners (MHQP) indicate there may be a disconnect between how clinicians are using the EHR and how patients are viewing the state of their care.

MHQP's 2007 Statewide Survey of Patient Experiences with their Primary Care Physician indicates that not all of the pistons are firing when it comes to how practitioners communicate EHR information to their patients:

✔ More than 1/3 of adult patients reported that their doctor did not always seem to know all the important information about their medical history.

✔ Forty percent of patients reported that their primary care physician was not always informed and up to date about care they received from specialists.

✔ Almost one-third of patients (or parents of child patients) reported they did not always receive test results from someone in the doctor's office.

The move to your EHR gives you an opportunity to open the lines of communication with your patients and really understand how they perceive the quality of their care. Ask open-ended questions frequently and you may find a clearer picture of how your patients feel about the care you provide.

Free Marketing — What Your Patients Should Tell Their Friends

Your patients have the potential to be some of your biggest and most vocal EHR champions.   Patients are not going to be writing thank you notes to you expressing how much they love your new EHR. It's just not going to happen. So, be aware of positive patient feedback to determine opportunities for patient marketing.

In your printed marketing materials, give your patients ideas on how to communicate your EHR benefits to their friends and families, such as the following points:

✔ My doctor uses an EHR to save my health records in electronic form — no more paper charts.

✔ EHRs are private, safe, and secure. The only people who can see my health information are me, my providers, and anyone I designate.

✔ The office staff scans any paper forms I bring in, such as my insurance cards or school health forms.

✔ I like it that my physician can print materials such as a summary of my visit or a list of recommended services (for example, shots or screenings I might need in the future).

✔ The EHR allows outside health professionals (specialists or pharmacists) to view my records to provide care.

✔ I can manage all of my prescriptions and refill orders online now. It's much faster and more efficient.

✔ I can request that my doctor send e-mails, instant messages, or automated phone messages to communicate important information (such as appointment reminders).

✔ My doctor can use the EHR to set up referrals to specialists on my behalf.

✔ I receive faster and more efficient service during office visits.

✔ My labs and test results are available faster and I can view them online.

✔ I can access my medical records from a home computer. No more calling in to have records faxed.

✔ I have online access to my child's health records (like immunizations) for easy printing and access. This is especially useful when I have to send records for school, daycare, and sports programs.

✔ I have access to my parents' healthcare records because I have been designated their caregiver.

Chapter 13

Surviving the Go-Live

*I*t's go-live time! This is the moment you and your fellow employees have been waiting for — time to see all of your hard work at EHR adoption and implementation come to fruition as you begin your new life in a paperless world. Every planning meeting, every visit with the vendor rep, and every moment you spent making sure all the EHR's bells and whistles worked are about to pay big dividends when you start to use the power of EHR to stream-line your workflows and provide more efficient care to your patients.

Go-live has its own unique set of challenges and opportunities for which you'll want to prepare. In this chapter, we provide a few checklists (for the "big day"), so you can make sure you and your practice are 100 percent ready for the excitement of going live.

Creating a Go-Live Timeframe

We present a lot of to-do's in this chapter. To keep your go-live on a steady schedule, create a go-live timeframe. Work backward from the go-live date, and schedule incremental dates to complete all your final preparations.

Doing so creates some excitement and buzz within the office, and helps instill confidence in your EHR leadership and system. A firm date says, "Yes, we are really doing this, and it's going to be a good thing."

Don't communicate the final go-live date until you have spent some time with the vendor, worked in the system, and are confident in your (and their) ability to meet the date. If you announce the go-live date and then have to change it, your stakeholders may lose confidence in the EHR.

Go-live no-go's

You don't want to host the go-live of an EHR during certain times of the year. Make sure to consider these important dates:

Holidays. A no-brainer, really.

Heavy travel time. Any time physicians or support staff are on the road for conferences, training, or vacations is a bad time to start working with the EHR.

Flu season. You'll be busy enough.

Big vendor meetings. You want the attention of your vendor and the vendor leadership, customer managers, and often support staff are not in the office a few times a year — during annual user-group meetings or large industry conferences. You'll want the full attention of your vendor leadership, account manager, and support team, so don't schedule your go-live while the team is out of the office.

Certain days of the week. It seems like a little detail, but Mondays and Fridays aren't the best. Opt for a Tuesday or a Wednesday if you can (Mondays are usually the busiest clinic days). This allows you a day or two to mentally prepare for the new system. If you start on a Friday, people will forget a fair amount by the time Monday comes. Give people a few days in a row to get in the swing of things.

Preparing for Go-Live

All the planning in the world can't always prepare you for every possible scenario, but you can make your life (and the lives of your employees) go a bit more smoothly if you have an idea of what to expect during the go-live. The go-live process, no doubt, will throw you some curve balls, but they won't hit you between the eyes as long as you can anticipate some of the more routine aspects of the process. By planning for the go-live, you reduce the chances for error that might slow down your practice's ability to complete a full-scale EHR migration.

Making sure everyone's ready to roll

Say it with us — people, processes, and technology. This is going to be your mantra when the time comes to prep for the go-live. There should be no doubt in your mind that your move to EHR is imminent; you just have to make sure everyone else is on board with the migration.

Work with your EHR planning committee to transition the group's functions into EHR management mode. Your committee members can help you assess the readiness of employees and infrastructure. Most importantly, your planning committee can help you gain and maintain the staff buy-in you need to make the move to EHR.

Depending on how early you create your go-live timeframe, you can make it as detailed as you like. Set some assessments of your readiness a few months in advance, starting 45–60 days prior to go-live. You can create a formal survey or assessment tool for the staff and clinicians to complete it or you can informally ask the questions as part of a pre–go-live check-in.

Everyone should be clear on the following points at least two months prior to go-live:

✔ The strategic importance of this project and the EHR.

✔ How this project aligns with the values of your practice.

✔ The benefits and challenges of this project.

✔ How this project and the EHR will have a positive impact.

✔ The responsibilities in terms of training, use of the EHR, and the overall success of the implementation.

✔ What roles and workflows are changing and what's staying the same.

✔ The necessary computer skills for the training and, ultimately, for the EHR use.

Review some key points around 30 days prior to go-live:

✔ The go-live date and what that means for the practice.

✔ The training and go-live support.

✔ The workflows that are changing.

✔ How to describe the project to patients and communicate patient benefits in terms of access to information, quality, and safety.

✔ How to successfully use the EHR to care for patients.

✔ How to access the system to practice using the EHR.

Everyone should be good on the following points two to three weeks prior to go-live:

✔ Knows the available functionality of the EHR.

✔ Has completed training and proficiency testing.

✔ Can access the system from the office and from home.

✔ Can successfully implement the EHR.

  • Knows where to access and retrieve clinical data in the EHR.

  • Can complete each patient visit.

As you anticipate the go-live date, here are some final topics to go over with staff:

- ✔ Where support resources are available, including tip sheets and job aids.

- ✔ Who/where to ask for support during go-live.

- ✔ Changes to policies and procedures for the practice.

- ✔ The required skills and the confidence to perform go-live critical activities to care for patients

Although that may seem like a lot of goals, timeframes, and benchmarks, assessing everyone's readiness at several points along the way results in greater understanding of the EHR by employees and helps you get ready for the big day — your go-live.

Determining your office readiness

You may find it helpful to create a personalized go-live assessment, not unlike the one you took part in during the initial phases of EHR planning. Your vendor will have some ideas about what to include in such an assessment, but if you wish to create a customized version in-house, you can divide your checklist into some major categories, starting with technical readiness for go-live. Think about some of the following technical issues:

- ✔ EHR accessibility for each user on every workstation

- ✔ Workstations have the ability to print (and print to the right location)

- ✔ Workstations are properly labeled

- ✔ Interfaces are thoroughly tested from both a technical and clinical standpoint

- ✔ System speed is responsive with no noticeable delays

- ✔ Downtime strategy is in place and everyone knows how to access critical patient information

- ✔ Network, hardware, and software support resource plan is in place

- ✔ All volume testing and performance evaluations are complete

- ✔ All support plans are documented (help desk, support for remote access, error tracking, and so on.)

Putting on the brakes

If you've done the proper planning and jumped through all the adoption and initial implementation hoops, then you should be geared up for go-live. However, be on the lookout for signs that might indicate you need to step back and take a brief time-out from the go-live proceedings. Here are some red flags to watch out for prior to go-live:

Staff resistance or lack of buy-in

Lack of funding

Lack of preliminary preparations

Unfinished interfaces

Incomplete system build or configuration

Incomplete testing

Too little training

Surprise obstacles

Unrealistic expectations

If any of these issues pop up, it may serve your practice well to spend a few extra weeks on addressing the issue preventing you from going live. Migrating to an EHR is a long-term proposition, so you want to do it right the first (hopefully, last) time.

You also have to assess your readiness in the areas of workflow design (and redesign). Consider whether you've taken these steps in anticipation of your go-live:

✔ Workflow procedures have been changed in preparation of go-live and have been documented in the training and support materials

✔ Workflows are in place for

- Office visits
- Phone calls
- Prescriptions
- Noting sensitive chart information
- Visit documentation
- Handling patients no longer served at your practice (moved or deceased)
- Referrals and hospital admissions
- Chart information requests
- Entering lab results or diagnostic information
- Downtime
- Incorporating paper documents or external documents into the EHR

Review interoffice protocols for how you will handle the actual documentation of workflows along with making sure the new and improved workflows are ready to be implemented. You want to be sure that you have a plan for keeping track of these new ways of conducting day-to-day business so that when it comes time to go-live, you have the appropriate documents available for quick reference.

If the system is not set up to meet your needs, the go-live won't go smoothly, or "go" at all. So, be sure you've cleared these hurdles:

- ✔ All users are active and privileges are assigned within the system
- ✔ Patient accounts are created and key information is preloaded into the EHR
- ✔ Passwords are activated
- ✔ Document views are created
- ✔ Customized content is created
- ✔ All document templates are created
- ✔ Encounter types are set up

Choosing a Go-Live Strategy

You can use a couple of strategies to go-live, and your choice depends largely on your comfort level with change. While moving through the adoption and implementation processes, you'll notice how everyone in the office is transitioning to the EHR environment. Are employees having trouble adjusting to the idea of using an all-electronic environment? Or, has everyone been trained and full of excitement and anticipation of moving to the twenty-first century?

If staff is having trouble adjusting to the idea of using the EHR, consider an incremental rollout strategy that phases in the implementation. For example, you could use the EHR for brand-new patients at first and slowly move into using it for long-time clients. You could use the EHR to only work on patients who fall into one of your managed (or "watch") groups. An incremental go-live can get you up and running, eventually, by easing the pace a bit.

If staff is ready and feeling confident, you should consider the "Big Bang" implementation method. In this case, the go-live occurs at one time — all recording functions and patient encounter types begin right away. There are no do-overs — you're up and running immediately. Because there's no time for reconsidering how you want to perform a specific function, you're invested in performing the tasks the way you've set them up. Table 13-1 details the pros and cons of each go-live scenario.

Table 13-1	Go-Live Scenario Pros and Cons	
Scenario Type	*Pros*	*Cons*
Incremental	Reduces element of surprise for employees	Overall training and implementation costs may be higher
	Spreads out costs of longer period of time	Benefits not realized as quickly
		Risk of failing to fully migrate to EHR documentation
	Lower chance for catastrophic project failure	
Big Bang	Shortens period of time in which you are using/accessing both paper AND electronic records	Higher risk of project failure
		Significant initial loss in productivity
	Faster achievement of EHR benefits	Higher chance for physician or staff rebellion if change is too drastic or swift
	Less chance of getting stuck in the implementation process and not achieving end goal of full migration	

There are pros and cons of each method of go-live; it really is up to you to determine what works best for your practice and patient population.

Completing Final Checks

When you determine that, in theory, you and the other practice employees are ready to commit to going live, you can begin to check the final implementation go forwards off your to-do list. While counting down the weeks and days to go-live, expect a bustle of activity in the office, ranging from final technology checks to the very important business of buying enough chocolate and caffeinated beverages to get everyone though the big day (or days).

Remember your EHR mantra — people, processes, technology — so you can be sure that you've laid the necessary groundwork in the days leading up to implementation. In the people category, host a few final meetings prior to go-live (yes, yes . . . *more* meetings) so you can answer final questions, review updated workflows, and build excitement for the go-live. Do a final headcount for who's been trained and who might need a refresher course. Generally, just do a lot of "checking in" pre–go-live to ensure that your employees are ready for the challenges ahead.

The same goes for your processes. If you answered all the readiness questions, you should have a final list of the changes in your workflows. Add another layer of process readiness at this point by making sure that implementation events are in place, such as modifying appointment times to account for any learning curves associated with EHR migration.

Work backward from your go-live date to schedule final implementation events. This can help you allow enough time for each specific event.

Do a final tech check by trying a dress rehearsal on the dummy patient accounts you created during training, running sample reports, making sure the hardware is working efficiently and correctly, and testing your backup protocols.

You can use the following checklist to make sure you haven't left anything out of the final go-live planning stage.

People

❑ All training complete and attendance confirmed

❑ Everyone has signed off on new EHR policies and workflows

❑ Morning staff have agreed to arrive 30 minutes to one hour early to prepare for first patients

❑ Everyone has had the opportunity to practice a dummy patient visit from start to finish, ask questions, and amend glitches

❑ Appointment times and employee schedules have been modified to account for go-live

❑ Patients who have appointments have been notified that your employees are implementing a new EHR, and you've asked for their patience during the transition

❑ Signage placed in and around office notifies patients of ongoing EHR implementation

❑ You've established a "go-live — free" zone in the office where employees can relax and grab a snack or soda

❑ Pep talk given to encourage and excite everyone

Processes

❑ New workflows established and communicated to employees

❑ Manuals set out at each workstation

❑ Login names, passwords, and procedures finalized

❑ Each workflow tested for accuracy

❑ Sample reports and forms printed to confirm accuracy

❑ Support procedures in place

❑ EHR champion(s) procedures confirmed

❑ Downtime procedures and forms in place

❑ Vendor rep and other support resources roles established

Technology

❑ System has been tested and documented

❑ System backups tested and validated

❑ Paper copies of all forms and templates available in case of system failure

❑ Computers, laptops, and peripherals tested

❑ Wireless hardware tested for connectivity

❑ Redundant lines tested (for ASP models only)

❑ System faxes and interfaces tested and working

❑ All devices are connected to printers and can print from the EHR system

Getting go-live support from peers and colleagues from other practices is a good idea. If you are part of a larger practice, and your clinic is going live first, get support from staff or physicians at other clinics that will be going live soon. Peers from other practices that are using the same EHR vendor can provide much needed support, too.

Managing the Go-Live

Eventually, you get to stop talking about going live and actually get down to business and do it. At the end of the day, remember that patient care comes first. If you focus on that, everything else will fall into place.

Getting your EHR off to the right start

On day one, you don't just waltz in, flip a switch, and hope for the best. Instead, you express guidance and calm nerves to make sure your employees are prepared for go-live. A pre–go-live meeting to walk everyone through the process one last time and answer questions may be helpful, too.

The go-live morning meeting is a great place to allow everyone to share their anxiety so you can address employees' fears and concerns.

Depending on your vendor and overall training strategy, you may elect to conduct some final training on the morning of go-live. This can serve as a final refresher course to make sure everyone remembers the new workflows and major functionalities of the EHR. Again, taking time to calm any jitters is never a bad idea.

When you open for business on go-live day, the months of hard work become a reality and you begin to serve patients by using the EHR. Follow these patient-related tips during the go-live and the weeks that follow:

- **Remember to tell patients that you're going live with a new EHR.** Patients are part of this journey, too.

- **Stay positive.** No one benefits if you display a negative outlook. Patients are concerned with their health issues, not whether you're using a new EHR.

- **Don't complain in front of patients.** You know that something won't go perfectly. Be prepared and try to reserve any negative comments about the go-live for after hours.

- **Have some talking points about patient benefits.** This is the patients' EHR migration, too; fill them in on some of the features that will help make their care experience more efficient and more user-friendly. We give you some talking points in Chapter 12.

So that you keep your sanity while getting through those first few patient visits on go-live day (and beyond), give yourself (and your employees) permission to move slowly and even make a few mistakes. We're human, and the EHR isn't going catch all your mistakes all the time. It's okay — really! Keep your cool by remembering a few first day tips:

- **You don't have to do everything in front of the patient.** This is why you built in extra time — so you and your employees can have more time between patients to enter information and practice new workflows.

- **You have the paper chart for key reference points.** Consider it your safety net.

- **Place your orders before a patient leaves.** This way, the patient is still in the office should you have follow-up questions.

- **Give patients a summary of their visit.** At a minimum, this usually involves demographic information, their current med list, allergies, reason for visit, any labs or studies you ordered, and any follow up information.

- **Complete your notes outside of the patient room.** Some people wait until lunch or after the clinic is closed for the day to catch up, but if you can, finish your notes before you go to the next patient. This is why you don't have a full schedule right now, so take advantage of it.

Another element of go-live is continuing to scan patient records. You likely have preloaded some core paper-based patient information, such as medications, allergies, and history elements, but some patient information may still be missing from the EHR. When you first see a patient after the go-live, you'll probably realize that some additional information should have been scanned and included in the EHR (maybe an EKG; an important note from a cardiology consult; or an old, but critical, lab result). Remember that all patient information is valuable because you never know when you might need it to help diagnose a condition. Use a sticky note or other tool to have the physician note any information that they want scanned into the EHR from the paper record.

Getting into an EHR routine

While the "new" wears off on your go-live experience, you and your employees begin to settle into a routine. After those first few patient visits using EHR are out of the way, everyone will feel a lot more confident about how they process patients and provide care in an electronic environment. Soon after, those pesky paper charts will be a thing of the past. First, you have to get through those initial weeks and months. Here are some tips to keep things rolling along:

- ✔ **First week**

  - Reduced schedule for everyone.

  - Remember that this is not just about the docs — it's about empowering all employees to use the EHR to provide a better quality of care. Even if the physicians, or at least a few, pick up the EHR quickly, you need everyone on the team to be functioning at a higher level before you start adding more patients to the schedule.

  - Allow time for abstracting information and scanning. Staff members are going to take longer to room a patient because they may be entering in a lot of information for the first time.

- ✔ **First Month**

  - Start increasing schedules after the first week. Some clinics slowly bring everyone to a full schedule at the same time. Others leave it up to the physician and their team. That way, if they're ready, they can get back to full productivity earlier.

  - Have a plan in place to wean physicians and staff off the paper charts for good and start implementing it now.

Remember the letters E-H-R. We know of one clinic that decided to allow the physicians to have the paper chart at the patient visit for the first three visits after go-live. After the first visit, the doctor would put an "E" on the chart; after the second visit, an "H"; and then an "R" at the third visit. The plan was to permanently retire the chart after spelling EHR. Employees soon realized that physicians started telling the staff that they didn't need the chart after the first visit. Having the chart made the providers feel more at ease, but they realized the EHR had the information they needed. This simple task provided enough of a safety net to help physicians make the jump to EHR without hanging onto the charts forever. Good thing, because estimates put the annual cost of maintaining and pulling charts at $4–$8 per patient. You want to start realizing those cost benefits sooner rather than later.

Many clinics reduce their schedule for the first week by 50 percent. Additionally, many practices do not schedule any major procedure visits or new patients. After a week or two, increase the schedule to 75 percent and then jump to a full schedule by the third or fourth week.

Remember to congratulate your team and yourself for braving these changes — new technology, new workflows, and new attitudes. Hand out compliments and provide a helping hand to anyone in the office who may be struggling with the go-live experience. After all, you're the resident EHR champion, so get out there and show everyone that you're committed to helping them achieve their goal of providing the best care experience to their patients.

Determining the Effects on Your Practice

When your practice acclimates to the world of EHR, you can chart the effects that the migration has had on your practice. Hopefully, the effects are positive for the most part. Although you may be spending most of your time making sure everything is working properly and everyone is using the EHR at full capacity, find time to note how the EHR is changing office life in terms of productivity, patients, and (no pun intended) patience.

Productivity

If everyone survives the go-live with few ramifications, their productivity should improve over time while they continue to master their EHR skills. You can look at productivity in two ways; both are important to you and your practice:

- ✔ **The number and types of patients that you see per day:** That's easy to gauge and you can adjust everyone's schedule over time to get back to 100 percent.

- ✔ **How much time everyone is spending documenting and working in the EHR:** Many clinicians spend lunch hour catching up or even end up working on charts from home.

Seeing the same number of patients as before doesn't mean that your office is back to full productivity. Capture how much time everyone is really working in the EHR and don't be satisfied until you and your staff are back and ahead of your baseline.

The reduced patient period passes eventually, and you begin to get a more accurate picture of how productive employees are using the new EHR. Hopefully, some of the EHR benefits that sold you on migrating will come to fruition as productivity ramps up:

✔ More time for patients; less time spent chasing down charts

✔ Entering information once and using automated forms to speed the process

✔ Less time spent deciphering handwriting

✔ More time for administrative staff to attend to billable tasks; less administrative burden

✔ Better accuracy in coding and billing; less time spent fixing mistakes

✔ Less time spent chasing down late reimbursements because of improper coding or missed information

✔ More information entered at the point of care; less time spent catching up on charting and paperwork

You probably won't return to full productivity as fast as you want. If you notice that productivity is not increasing how you hoped, find out why. Perhaps you've experienced technical difficulties that prevented staff from utilizing the fullest EHR functionality. Maybe the learning curve is simply leveling out slower than you wanted. Keep communicating with employees and physicians so you can determine the cause of any slowed productivity.

Patients

Your patients are affected by the EHR migration, too. Although some patients may visit you only once or twice a year, ultimately, they're still the beneficiaries of what EHR has to offer. Better quality of care, more efficient visits, improved ways to actively participate in their own health care management — these should have, if all goes well, a positive effect on your patients.

When you see patients for return visits post–go-live, ask them about their experience with your new setup. Do they feel they are receiving better (or, at the very least, good) care? Do they see a change in how quickly their check-in and intake processes proceed? Have they experienced any glitches with prescriptions or services rendered outside your office?

Aside from verbally communicating your questions, you might want to consider handing out a simple questionnaire after their first EHR experience. Alternatively, you can set up a phone-based or online survey that can automatically chart and provide responses on a regular basis. If you're implementing a patient portal (see Chapter 15), you can use those tools to capture patient satisfaction information, too.

Patience

The office atmosphere can be greatly affected by how everyone adapts to the EHR and responds to the stress associated with such a global change. For example, employee fuses that are a bit short because something isn't going right with the go-live can have lasting effects on interoffice relationships. Don't let the temporary stresses of go-live overshadow the progress everyone has made with the EHR implementation.

Check attitudes weekly by initiating casual conversations around the office, observing how employees respond when a glitch occurs, and reading the employees' patience during staff meetings.

Remind employees that the go-live phase (and the weeks that follow) is no time to play office politics. If someone is having an issue related to the go-live, encourage him or her to mention it so you can help find a solution. Create opportunities for everyone to communicate their suggestions, complaints, and general comments.

Evaluating Your System Post–Go-Live

A few weeks or months after your go-live when the EHR is just another part of practice life, you start to note patterns, benefits, and overall quality of service that you're providing with the electronic platform. To get the most accurate picture of how the EHR is working out for you after the go-live, evaluate the following:

- ✔ **People:** Your employees are your most important resource. Watch for an unhappy person (especially a physician) who can derail all the hard work you and your staff have put in to the EHR implementation. Remember that go-live is stressful, tempers can flare, and anxiety may be prevalent. So, take the temperature of the staff regularly. Provide a room or an area where people can relax for a minute or two, and have food and drink available.

- ✔ **Issue resolution:** Follow your issue resolution process (you do have one, right?). Track the issues, who is reporting them, who needs to fix them, and the resolution.

Some measurements won't start right at go-live but the following key information can help you track your go-live metrics:

- ✔ **Use**
  - Number of concurrent users
  - Total users (ideally, this is everyone in the clinic)

- Number of orders placed by physicians and number of physicians placing orders (ideally, all of them)

✔ **Verbal orders**

- Number of completed charts and average time to complete a chart

✔ **IT**

- Number of outstanding issues

- Number of resolved issues

- Average time for issue resolution by category

✔ **Patient**

- Number of patients seen

- Number of patients receiving a summary from their visit

✔ **Cost**

- Level of Service

- Charge capture for procedures, supplies, and so on.

Use the metrics you evaluate to create a list of go-forwards for your post–go-live life, including additional training you want to offer employees, communications with outside entities you wish to prioritize, and updates or upgrades you wish to add to the EHR system. Look at Chapter 16 to see more ways to continually improve your EHR.

Part IV
Optimizing and Improving Your EHR

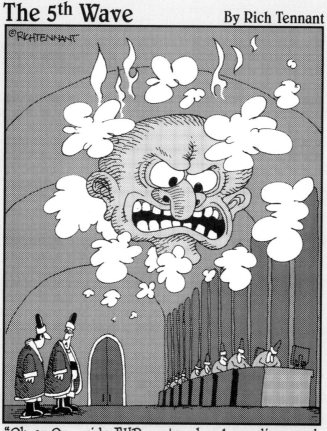

The 5th Wave   By Rich Tennant

"Oh, an Oz—wide EHR system has been discussed, but it's not as impressive as the giant, floating, disembodied head of the Wizard keeping an eye on everything."

In this part . . .

This part shows you how to make the most of the EHR experience. Chapter 14 focuses on managing groups of patients, and Chapter 15 gives you plenty of tips for helping patients participate in their own care management. Chapter 16 is a guidebook of sorts, helping you clear the way for tweaking and updating the EHR system as time marches on.

Chapter 14

Keeping Your Patients Healthy with an EHR

*Y*ou're probably pretty psyched about all the ways EHR will benefit you and your practice staff. Less paper, greater efficiency, and streamlined workflows are all huge bonuses. Now, though, it's time to think about some ways EHR can benefit your patients. Aside from faster service and features, such as electronic prescribing (which, admit it, is pretty cool), another big payoff for patients is better health. When you use an EHR, you increase your ability to provide directed patient care that will help both you and your patients manage healthcare needs in a way that promotes long-term health benefits.

The key term in this chapter is *care management,* which is simply the coordination of healthcare services to meet the needs of an individual or a population of patients. Not unlike *care coordination* (which is more about the individual steps than the overall concept or plan), care management encompasses an umbrella process that reviews, plans, implements, coordinates, tracks, and evaluates functions and services to manage healthcare needs. Figure 14-1 shows how EHR care management fits with some of the other functions of the clinical setting.

When setting up your plans for care management, think about your practice's quality goals, which may include such topics as efficiency, safety, effectiveness, patient-centered focus, and timely delivery of services (or anything else you want to add to your goal laundry list). Then, you can use these goals and concepts surrounding care management to help improve your patients' health and quality of life. By focusing on two vital components of your patient population, you can cover a lot of ground and use your EHR to do it. With EHR, you can manage large patient groups and provide care for patients with chronic diseases or conditions.

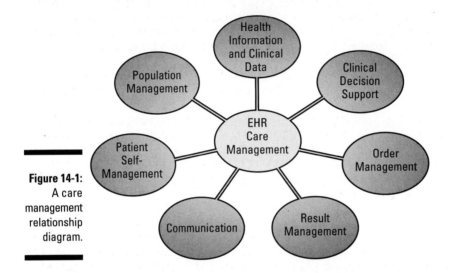

Figure 14-1:
A care
management
relationship
diagram.

Managing Large Groups of Patients

When you start to use an EHR, you're generally focused on a single patient. But as you start to get comfortable with your new tools, the greatest power lies not in managing one patient but looking at whole groups of patients. You can take the knowledge you gain from one patient and use it to manage care for an entire population of patients. EHRs can perform many functions and support workflows that help you keep track of all sorts of patient groups from those with chronic illnesses or recurring conditions to those whom you classify by subjects, such as age or family history.

Benefits associated with managing an entire population of patients include

- ✔ Timelier tracking of patients
- ✔ Stronger coordination of care
- ✔ Ability to indentify patients who are overdue on their follow-up visits and tasks
- ✔ Clearer feedback provided to care team
- ✔ Ability to assign patients to appropriate risk groups to foster more directed care management

Of course, these benefits aren't magically bestowed upon your practice as soon as you go-live. You have to set up your system to accommodate group management functions (such as patient registries, for example) and work with your vendor rep to make sure your system offers the features and functionalities that make group care management possible. Using standards-based EHRs that include clinical decision support and registry functionality can support reporting, tracking, and managing patients by condition, problem, or diagnosis. Your EHR can be a useful tool in determining the effectiveness of treatment or health of your practice's patient population.

Not all EHR systems can aggregate individual data, so confirm with your vendor that yours does and find out how it works prior to implementation.

Just because you have the ability to manage care on a wider scale doesn't mean that you should forgo personal service to individual patients. What managing patients based on group characteristics means is that you can offer care solutions based on trends that you notice while managing the entire patient population. By seeing the big picture, you can provide better service and more direct care to individual patients.

Start off by setting up your system to identify patient groups. After you clear that hurdle, you can set up the system to chart processes and outcomes and provide feedback. Then you can set your sights on planning services for each patient group. Once you get started, it really is fun to see how each patient group differs in terms of characteristics, care approaches, and progress. If you've never been able to manage groups because there was no efficient way to track their progress (aside from more charts), now is your opportunity to really change the way you provide care and revolutionize the way you interact with specific patient populations.

Identifying patient groups with registries

Step one in the group management journey is to identify patient groups and set up registries. After all, how will you know what services and care to offer if you don't know whom it's for? Registries in combination with clinical decision support can use symptoms, other diagnoses, and labs to identify patients who may have a disease before you or someone in your practice has diagnosed them. Setting up patient registries can also help you track outcomes and ongoing progress, look at your treatment methods, and make adjustments across an entire population (and meet some requirements of Meaningful Use, too).

Patient group registries aren't the complete answer to all your clinical questions. You still have to enter and pull data correctly. Getting the right data entered is crucial because you don't want to leave patients off the registry. Your information capture needs to consist of structured data and not just a text-based note. Most EHRs can't mine free text information and pull out salient details, but the use of natural language processing is likely to come in future products. Natural language processing can convert free text into coded information.

While you're designing and using your EHR to capture information:

- ✔ **Identify key information that you want to report on and monitor.** This may include HgbA1C results for patient with diabetes, documentation that you completed a foot exam, or acknowledgment that a patient had her mammogram performed. Be sure to include the following:

  - Any quality measures that you need to report for PQRI, CMS, or any internal program.

  - All key Clinical Quality Measures (CQM) from the Meaningful Use criteria that you will be reporting.

- ✔ **Work with your vendor.** Make sure your EHR includes all the structured data fields you need to capture the information you want to track.

- ✔ **Decide whether you want to require staff or other physicians to document the information.** Many EHRs have functionality that requires end users to complete certain information that's required.

  - Educate and obtain "buy in" from your practice when implementing required data fields as it can create frustration when users are forced to enter data that they don't feel is crucial.

- ✔ **Develop the necessary workflow to capture the right information.** Be sure your workflows contain

  - A process to document information, such as a colonoscopy or mammogram report, from an outside source.

  - The optimal method and person to enter information into the EHR. Sometimes it may be the physician, but it also may be appropriate for a nurse or other staff member to capture the result received for a patient.

- ✔ **Train and support.** All end users need to know the new workflow.

- ✔ **Run reports and follow up on the findings.** Confirm that your information is correct and not a result of someone entering the information incorrectly.

Your best bet is to capture patient data correctly the first time. This seems obvious, right? The way you "enter" information is not always the way you want to "view" information — so this means that you need to consider the views of information you may want when deciding how to enter data. If you don't identify the right information before you go-live, changing bad documentation habits or capturing requisite information going forward is difficult.

Work with the vendor to set up patient registry groups that you identify by certain characteristics. For the purposes of offering care in a clinical setting, set up groups based on risk or condition, which your EHR can stratify by using statistical data collected at the time of patient check-in. This way, though each individual patient has slightly different needs and outcomes, you can initialize their care options based on some common group features. For example, you could set up patient groups based upon conditions or diagnoses for those at risk for

- Coronary artery disease
- Heart failure
- Diabetes
- Stroke
- Cancer
- Asthma
- Depression
- Hypertension

You can also identify patient groups by conditions, such as

- Allergies
- Autoimmune disorders (such as lupus)
- Addictions
- Hormone disorders (hyperthyroidism, Addison's disease, Cushing's disease)
- Recurring infections
- Mental health issues

Other patient groups may include

- Certain medications
- Preventative care
- Wellness management

Not every patient will fall into one of the categories you designate because they haven't been identified as members of a high-risk category or as having a chronic condition. But you can work with that, too, by making non-group status a group and monitoring for status changes. That is, when a patient doesn't fall into a designated group, your EHR can monitor that patient's file for any changes in health status.

One of the lead identifiers of your patient groups will be *overdue* patients — patients who are overdue for specific tests or procedures. By incorporating specific timeframe requirements for care benchmarks, your EHR system can red flag any patients who haven't had them. Consider it your group care management flare gun, shooting out a spark every time a patient is overdue for a test or procedure.

Ask your vendor rep if you can set up patient group lists to notify you of any global changes to a patient's health status that might remove them from that particular group. If, for example, Mrs. Jones experiences a significant weight loss and reverses her pre-diabetes, does your EHR have the ability to move her out of the pre-diabetes group or notify you that she no longer fits the criteria for the group?

Planning and offering services and interventions

After you identify patient groups, you can then use that population segmentation (a very official way to say "groups") to set up various services and interventions to help your staff and members of that patient group manage their care.

This is really a "blue sky" moment for your practice because the possibilities for group care can be endless, especially when it's facilitated by an EHR. Work with your transition team and your vendor rep to think of useful ways to step up the quality of the care you offer to these groups. Run reports and look at which patient statuses are populating your registry.

Many of your patients with chronic diseases may not come in as often as they should. Disease registries and associated decision support tools can help provide triggers and tools to identify patients who need to come in. Perhaps you want to make educational intervention a priority. Or maybe you want to make sure the basic needs and requirements of a group are covered, such as regular testing or biannual appointments to screen for new complications. Registries in combination with clinical decision support can be used to identify patients based on symptoms or other diagnoses and labs, which may diagnose a patient's disease before you or someone in your practice.

It's your show, really, so set up your care benchmarks in a prioritized matrix that allows you to put the care requirements you deem most important first. Here are some of the useful tasks you can set up using the EHR for group management:

✔ Activate patients who are overdue for preventive screenings using e-mail or phone reminders

✔ Monitor medication adherence

✔ Monitor patients on a certain medication

✔ Set up clinical intervention notes or reminders for your staff

✔ Chart test results

✔ Create a calendar or to-do list for the patient

✔ Provide tools for patient self-management

✔ Set up group visits to address common issues and build camaraderie between patients with similar conditions

✔ Segment patient population to administer specialized educational interventions

- Alerts and reminders

- Mailing or e-mailing of educational materials

- Notifications about new drugs

- E-mail blast about new research findings

When you go-live, you may not have this information entered or preloaded in the EHR; therefore, your reports won't be accurate. So make sure during your preloading processes, you capture this vital information in a structured, coded format (such as problem list, medication list, allergies list, lab values) versus scanned into the EHR or as a text-based note. If you miss important information during preloading, enter it during the next patient visit — if the relevant information is documented in a free text field, the EHR can't report on it or support identification of a patient group based upon that data.

Not all of these newly created group care processes and interventions have to be obvious to your patient. You can also set up processes that are apparent only to your staff to provide seamless care to all patients. For example, if you want to create a specific time during the day that you only see one group of patients, you can do that. Or, perhaps you want to be sure that the primary physician performs all the face-to-face appointments with a specific group instead of assigning those patients to the nurse practitioner. You can do that! And your EHR can help. Figure 14-2 shows how you can incorporate these group care processes into your workflow.

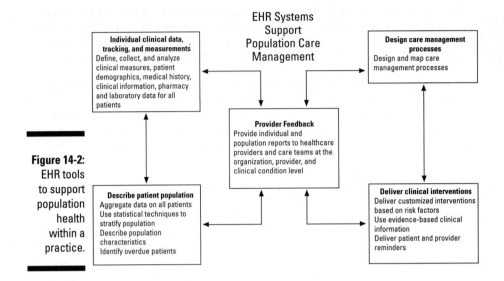

Figure 14-2:
EHR tools
to support
population
health
within a
practice.

Reporting processes and outcomes

All of this specialized group care management means a lot more to
your practice and to your patients in the long run if you can chart and
report how your efforts are working for both your patients and the
overall management style of your practice. Creating reports is an easy
way to track your progress.

You can set up the EHR to run reports on just about anything related
to group care management. You can find out the percentage of patients
who show up for specific appointment types, how many patients
required changes in medications over a period, what type of diagnostic
imaging was most used in each group, and a host of other information.

Vendors will have reports that you won't have to configure, but you'll
want to make sure that you're capturing necessary information to populate the report. You can also ask how to develop your own reports.
Sometimes the vendors will do this for you — it might be an extra
charge or you can negotiate a certain number be done per year. Match
these reports with your quality goals and any financial incentives you
might have. You may even tie a bonus payment for providers to their
patient outcomes.

You can count on the EHR to have the capacity to run a report for just about anything you want to know as long as the information is entered in the system. If the EHR doesn't run a report you need, tell your vendor rep. Maybe your vendor can integrate that feature into your EHR on the next upgrade cycle.

You can use the EHR to obtain patient profiles for each group, providing you with a glimpse into what the "typical" patient looks like for that particular condition. This comes in handy when you are reporting to outside specialists or agencies so they may plan appropriate responses to patient groups. You can also use these profiles to assist patients within the group with setting up personal care goals and plans.

For example, say you have statistical information provided by your EHR to create a profile of the average diabetic patient under the age of 40. Perhaps what you find is that patients with this profile typically have a BMI of over 35 and a sedentary lifestyle (both contribute to the condition). You can relay that information to your patients to spark a discussion about action plans related to healthy weight loss, which has the potential to lower their glucose numbers and allow them to better control their condition (or potentially reverse diabetes altogether). Because the common thread you see for this particular group is age (under 40) and weight, you can create educational materials that show them how to lower their BMI, lose at least 10 percent of their body weight, incorporate exercise, and make healthy eating choices.

Got group?

One way you can manage group care more efficiently is to use your EHR to coordinate group visits. These are not meant to replace the standard office visit, but are considered extensions of the traditional visit that can help you answer common questions and allow for patients to meet and coordinate care ideas with patients like them. By using group visits, your practice can

✔ Lower instances of patient hospital admissions and length of stay

✔ Reserve a majority of individual visits for subspecialty issues

✔ Increase patient satisfaction

✔ Allow for social interaction among patients with similar needs

✔ Open more time to discuss medication issues, self-management support, and specialty services that may be appropriate for group members

✔ Discuss self-management progress and adherence to treatment

✔ Assess global needs

✔ Distribute educational information more efficiently

✔ Provide a forum for patients to discuss the emotional aspects of their care needs

Adding these kinds of appointments to the mix can greatly increase your face time with patients while offering them the benefit of meeting others in a similar care situation.

Providing feedback

You can also set up group management features to provide more detailed feedback to other healthcare providers at the organizational, provider, and clinical conditions level. Using your EHR to provide group care feedback to your staff as well as specialists and providers outside the office or clinical setting helps facilitate the availability, timeliness, and accuracy of messages among these groups.

The goal here, for both you and colleagues outside the office, is to interact with each other, open your communications (which you should be doing anyway thanks to the EHR), and work together to provide solutions for the groups you manage. This helps you coordinate any care services that you offer as the result of a referral or diagnostic need, and establish clear roles and responsibilities for employee teams in your office and colleagues with whom you work outside the office. By sharing feedback and coordinating your efforts, you can do a more efficient job of anticipating patient needs and providing long-term care management solutions.

Managing Patients' Chronic Diseases

Managing groups of patients is certainly beneficial to your practice and your patients because it helps you and your practice's employees envision what the care model can look like for an entire patient population. But eventually you will want to drill down your care management efforts to the individual patient. Not that you aren't doing that already — we certainly hope you're making each individual patient a priority! But particularly in the case of patients with chronic conditions, individualized care management service is a vital component of their overall healthcare picture. Your EHR can help you streamline the workflows associated with chronic disease management and improve the way you manage care for these patients.

Chronic illnesses are no joke. Some statistics report that more than 90 million Americans experience at least one chronic illness, leading to 7 of every 10 deaths in the United States. Not only do these numbers affect the survival rate of the country's population; they also lead to increased healthcare costs and are responsible for 75 percent of total national healthcare expenditures.

Virtually all growth in Medicare expenditures can be attributed to about one-half of the beneficiaries that are suffer from a combination of chronic illnesses.

You have a choice to make about chronic disease management. You can solely use the EHR, you can go with chronic disease management (CDM) tools, or you can use a combination of both. EHRs are more complex and have disease management tools as part of their functionality, while CDM tools may be used as a precursor to an EHR or in conjunction with an EHR, depending on its functionality. CDM tools are population-based, disease-specific tools that are not complete EHRs or medical records. CDMs and EHRs are similar in that they use evidence-based guidelines to manage patients, and they use tools to track and engage patients.

EHR patient and disease management tools include

✔ **Registries:** List of patients with the same disease or same characteristics. Most common registries are for asthma, diabetes, and heart failure.

✔ **Clinical reports:** Compiled data based on criteria that show patient results and outcomes.

✔ **Assessment tools:** Patient self-assessment and staff-delivered assessments.

✔ **Evidence-based content:** Examples include order sets and care plans.

✔ **Patient portal:** Electronic means for patient to receive information about their care and ideally input their own information, too.

✔ **Decision support:** Rules and alerts that can trigger actions from different care team members. For example, sending a letter to a patient to schedule an appointment or submit his or her latest glucometer readings.

✔ **Communication tools:** Means to update and involve other care team members and the patient in ongoing activities.

✔ **Education materials:** Specific tools to inform patients about their disease process, resources to research the disease, or additional support groups.

All of these tools can help your practice improve its group care, and practitioners can set up a combination of these tools to customize their group care management plan.

Roles and responsibilities

Care management doesn't deliver itself; it requires people. Your staff has to maneuver many moving parts and many active roles to ensure the group management effort is coordinated, cost-effective, and beneficial to patients.

At the top of your care management food chain is the physician. In this context, doctors help guide and lead the care management efforts, though the majority of work is be done by the team and the patient. The physician helps to confirm that care guidelines and the overall plan are evidenced-based (and continue to be when evidence and recommendations change). If you think of disease management as an extension of the physician practice, you can see how vital it is to have someone championing those efforts and making sure that the quality of your group management is as high as the quality of the individualized care your practice provides.

Next, the group care management team consists of educators, nurses, and case managers. Depending on the setup and culture of your practice, these roles can be played by people who aren't employed by just one practice, but instead are shared between practices. This comes in handy if, say, you want to monitor a group based on mental health needs, but your practice doesn't have someone on staff with a wide-reaching knowledge in that area. In this case, you could work in conjunction with a mental health practitioner outside your office to provide optimal care to these patients.

EHR provides a great tool for multiple stakeholders to track and document their involvement with a patient. Ideally, different decision support tools can be triggered for different roles. For example, the case manager could get an alert to call a patient if the patient hasn't scheduled his three-month diabetes follow-up. The patient gets the reminder, and the physician doesn't have to get involved unnecessarily.

Members of the care team can work with the patient on goal planning and goal documentation. If you connect your EHR to a patient portal, patients can track their goals and progress electronically. Care team members can also provide support to patients by following up on their care "to-do" lists, offering educational materials as needed, and monitoring developments in research and news related to common conditions.

Exploring the patient centered medical home (PCMH)

The patient centered medical home (also referred to as PCMH or simply, "medical home") originated in the pediatrics setting to develop a model for care that is "accessible, continuous, comprehensive, family-centered, coordinated, compassionate, and culturally effective to all children and youth, including those with special health care needs." The medical home concept was soon adapted in primary care as a model of care where all care givers work in partnership with the patient and the patient's family. Health information technology plays a role with patient registries, EHRs, HIEs, and other means to identify and manage patients. Although the concept of the medical home has been around for some time, there has been resurgence in the initiative at the local and national levels. More and more practices are embracing the idea and some funding is available for implementation from employers, health plans, and national organizations.

PCMHs provide a means to deliver comprehensive care to all patients by involving the physician, the team, the patient, and other caregivers. The team is directed by the physician, but the entire office participates in the care of the patient. Thus, the "patient-centered" portion of the name. Care is coordinated across sites including ambulatory practices, the hospital, and the patient home.

Obviously, the patient is a vital member of the care group. After all, you wouldn't have anything to manage without the patient! Because patients have the most at stake of anyone involved in care management, they have to be active participants to reap the benefits of everyone else's efforts. Here is where your EHR comes in very handy. Patients can use patient portals to enter key information about the status of their health conditions, pull educational information, and track their latest lab or test results.

Many health plans offer services based on results of a patient survey or questionnaire. Health coaching is one of those services, in which a patient is assigned a coach who communicates with the patient online or via phone interview on a regular basis about any health concerns. Health coaches can make suggestions for self-care and follow up with the patient on a regular basis to see whether his or her care goals are being met.

Health plans can work with physicians to improve reimbursement or overall management, while remaining in the background of the care management process. Ideally, health plans should provide assistance and not be seen as a burden.

Focusing on outcomes

The good news is that healthcare IT, EHRs particularly, can improve the quality of care you provide to patients with chronic conditions. Many AHRQ-funded projects have found that by incorporating EHRs or other healthcare IT systems, practitioners can support improvements in outcomes for the chronically ill.

You can use the data you collect from your EHRs group management features to create outcome scenarios for individuals. Generally, for all of your patients with chronic conditions, you can focus on the following outcomes:

✔ **Physical**

- Increased energy

- Increased activity levels

- Improved overall quality of life

- Better symptom management

- Increased self-efficacy

- Less physical discomfort

✔ **Emotional**

- Fewer social limitations

- Psychological well-being

- Less anxiety or depressed moods
- Mental stress management

✔ **Clinical and Operational**

- Improved partnership with physician
- Improvement in self-rated health status
- Lower healthcare costs
- Fewer clinical visits
- Fewer hospital stays
- Open communication with physician
- Fewer ER visits

A big benefit of using the EHR to manage chronic conditions is, of course, financial. Your practice can earn financial incentives for managing patients differently through the use of care groups. Meaningful Use; global payments; readmission rates; and incentives from health plans, the government, and quality organizations are all tied to how your practice successfully manages groups. You receive money for upping your care management ante, but you can save money, too. EHRs can help you lower the costs associated with treating chronically ill patients, which saves your practice, your patients, and health plans a ton of cash.

Setting up a care management project

You can always set up your care management model on a trial basis and then collect and analyze the data to review the results before opting out or amending how the model is organized. Set a timeframe for your chronic care management trial run, stick to it, and debrief to find out what you might want to do differently long term.

The CMS provides some examples of care management projects that yielded positive results. One project that took place in three states used in-home remote monitoring of chronically ill patients. The devices transmitted data about vitals and weight. When a change in the patient's health occurred, the system alerted the patient and his or her providers, who were able to review the data and respond if any action was required. This system ultimately resulted in fewer trips to the ER and less time spent in a hospital. Additionally, patients reported that the system increased their confidence in their abilities to self-manage, and occurrences of medication usage errors lowered.

Providing integrated services

After you set some initial outcome goals for patients with identified chronic conditions, you can work with your staff to provide integrated services to manage their care. This is the "action" of your action plan. To use the EHR in conjunction with your care management goals and outcomes for chronically ill patients, work with your vendor rep to integrate the EHR system into your workflows. This will, in the long run, reduce the time and effort it takes clinicians to receive care recommendations from the system and put them into action. When you redesign your practice workflows (see Chapter 8), map the steps involved in your care management activities and integrate those into your new workflows, too.

Your EHR should have critical care management functions. Ask your vendor rep to make sure your system is set up to aggregate data, pull reports based on condition characteristics, and identify populations.

The services you provide for the management of chronic conditions and diseases depend entirely on what types of chronic conditions exist within your overall patient population. Generally, you can expect to offer these integrated services:

- ✔ Automatic appointment reminders
- ✔ Automatic reminders for diagnostic testing and preventive services
- ✔ Clinical decision support
- ✔ Educational materials including personalized reports, self-management templates, research findings, and lists of patient action items
- ✔ Support care coordination
- ✔ Delivery of patient-centered services

To illustrate how you can set up these integrated services, consider automatic reminders. You can set up the EHR to create a list of your practice's patients with a particular chronic disease, use that list to track key measures, and remind you and your staff automatically when patients need certain labs and preventive services. You can set up the EHR to make these lists and reminders available to anyone on your staff (including nurses, medical assistants, and administrative staff) with minimal training. For example, you can set up the EHR to notify you if the date of a diabetic patient's last A1C is more than 90 days ago. When that happens, the EHR turns the date cell yellow as a warning; if more than 180 days have passed, the date field turns red. Or, you can set up the date field to change colors if a patient's A1C is outside of the normal range. Visual cues allow staff members to scan the worksheet and quickly identify which patients are due for which service.

Reporting data

To manage patient groups successfully, you have to keep lines of communication wide open, starting with your care team. The team must create a means for patients to respond to and initiate care-related communications.

The push to communicate puts more responsibility on the shoulders of your care team to develop the workflow and messaging tools they want to use to interface with patients. Typically, the physician is updated but doesn't have to perform the majority of the communication tasks.

You have several ways to inform your patients about their care management. You can go traditional, using snail mail or phone. Or, you can use your EHR's communication features to help you generate automatic letters and calls, send e-mail, or send secure messages to a patient portal. No matter what method you choose to deliver information, make sure to get patient consent before initiating communication. Also, depending on the patient's age or mental capacity, you may want to provide proxy access for a parent or caregiver.

A useful aspect of the EHR that your care team can make wide use of for care management is the EHR's reminders and alerts. Again, the responsibility to create the parameters for how your practice uses alerts, what triggers alerts, and who receives alerts (nurse, case manager, physician, or patient) is on the care team.

If your team is a bit unsure of how best to use alerts, start with a few and increase the volume and complexity over time. However, monitor the utility of alerts — you don't want to cause "alert fatigue" where too many alerts fire and are not noticed or disregarded because they are a nuisance.

You have to work with your care team and patients, and report data to other entities when appropriate. By reporting data (such as quality indicators) to colleagues, specialists, and healthcare organizations, you improve quality and efficacy of the care you provide, which then benefits your chronic patients.

Set up your EHR to capture quality data during all patient encounters, including ones that involve diagnostic activities, and generate reports. For example, you can set up the EHR to identify patients whose diabetes isn't under control. Then, using the reports your EHR generates, your staff can call patients to provide education and support in management of their diabetes, which should allow your patients to improve their health status and develop skills to control their diabetes on their own.

Building an Accountable Care Organization (ACO)

Recently, the buzz surrounding the "medical home" has given way to the Accountable Care Organization (ACO), which has been touted as a promising model for health reform. New laws introduced in 2010 include funding of Medicare pilot programs to facilitate controlling the costs of Medicare. The ACO model is based on three design principles:

✔ Provider-led organizations are collectively accountable for a defined population of patients

✔ Payment reform that rewards quality improvements, contains costs, and avoids financial risks

✔ Performance measurement including patient experience data, clinical process, and outcome measures

EHRs, HIE, and patient registry functionality can be instrumental tools in identifying high-risk patients who need increased monitoring and management. Patient portals and PHRs can support patient access to their EHR information and work with care management, preventive care, and wellness tools that support the ACO model. Project data from CMS ACO demonstration sites is still being reviewed, but preliminary findings seem to indicate that mature electronic health record systems and health information exchange capabilities contributed to the success of five of the ten ACO demonstration sites funded by CMS.

Any time you can report data, whether it is to your in-house staff or to a national organization like CMS, you have the opportunity to share information that can improve how you conduct day-to-day interactions and encounters with chronically ill patients and increase patients' ability to manage their conditions. The circle analogy holds true — as long as the data is generated and shared among stakeholders, you can offer appropriate services and patients can achieve outcomes that improve their health status and quality of life. Each feeds into the other; you need all of these chronic care management participants involved to keep your patients healthy.

Chapter 15

Directing Patient Access and Communication

*I*t's time for you to use that EHR to show *and* tell your patients about what is going on with their care on a regular basis. The way you can do that is through providing patients with access to their personal health information (PHI) and offering them tools to communicate with your practice outside the clinical setting. By using a few patient communication tools, you can enhance (not replace) the face-to-face care you provide each day.

EHR offers structured and form-based tools, which can guide or limit the content of a patient's query to provide quicker routing of queries and increase workflow efficiency. Additionally, EHR-based communication tools typically offer stronger security features than standard e-mail, so you can put your mind (and your patients') at ease. All you have to do is decide what information you want to communicate with patients, the methods you want to use, and how much access you want to provide.

Giving Patients Appropriate Information Access

The type of care you provide greatly affects how you view patient communications. With an EHR, it's important for you to step up your efforts to provide *patient-centered care*. Your practice treats patients as partners in their care, not merely consumers of your services. By using patient-centered care, your practice is involving patients in the planning and management of their care and encouraging them to take responsibility for their own healthcare management.

With the new healthcare revolution in the United States, patients are more interested than ever in participating in the management of their healthcare. According to a recent Harris poll, 67 percent of patients said they would like to receive results online. Seventy-four percent would like to communicate via e-mail, and 77 percent would like to receive visit reminders via e-mail. Additionally, the majority said that the use of an EHR and the ability to connect via e-mail would influence their choice of physicians. Demand for access to information is obviously high among the patient population. Mega healthcare organization Kaiser Permanente's CEO reports they have nearly 9 million e-visits per year. That's a significant number, and one you shouldn't ignore. If you build the EHR communications portals, they will come!

Not only are patients interested in accessing records online for convenience, patients need to communicate online for better self-management. The need for increased patient-centered care is on the rise. Patients left unchecked after receiving care instructions or medications from their physician are more likely to misunderstand their care instructions or misuse medications.

Some clinical reports indicate that between 40 and 50 percent of patients with diabetes do not follow their established medication regimens, which can result in frequent clinical visits, increased hospitalization, and increased care costs down the road.

We're not saying that patients go completely off the rails with their self-care the moment they leave your practice. However, the more you can involve patients in the management of their own care, the better results they'll have with managing everyday healthcare issues and chronic disease management concerns. Your EHR is the gateway to making that possible.

Deciding what to share

You have to determine what kind of information you want to share with your patients. What you want your patients to know can drive your selection of delivery method. For example, you probably wouldn't want to deliver sensitive test results via instant message. IM may be fine for casual administrative reminders ("Hey! Your appointment is tomorrow!"), but not for telling a patient she has cancer. Take care to set parameters for the types of information you communicate in electronic form.

Table 15-1 gives you a view of potential patient communication topics.

Table 15-1	Possible Patient Communication Topics		
Administrative Needs and Tasks	**Prescriptions**	**Clinical Issues**	**Caregiver Questions and Concerns**
Appointment reminders	Reminders	Lab tests or diagnostic results that aren't life threatening	Communication with parents about child's healthcare needs, immunizations, and appointments
Registration	Refills	Immunization records and updates	Communication with adult children caring for an elderly parent (as long as consent is provided)
Billing issues or questions	Drug event or allergy questions	Allergy questions or recommendations	Educational materials
Insurance claims	Drug interaction updates	Action required after test results	Diagnosis-specific information
Coverage denials	Patient questions about medication instructions	Tracking of recurring test results	
Requests for information	Co-pays and coverage	Online consultations	
Visit reports	New medications	E-visits	
History	Medication changes	Questions about a condition	
Educational materials		Queries about basic symptoms	
		Problem lists	

You can create a similar listing of patient communication topics for your own practice so you can quickly see what information you want to share and decide how you want to share it. List potential questions or issues with each type of communication message, too. Consider how you will share the following information electronically:

- ✔ **Lab results:** When will you release results? Will the provider review everything before the results publish to the portal? Will results release automatically after a certain amount of time (for example, normal results immediately and abnormal results after 48 hours)?

- ✔ **Schedule:** Schedule appointments or at least request an appointment.

- ✔ **Medications:** Add new medications including other prescriptions, over the counter medications, and herbal remedies.

- ✔ **Problem list:** Will you include all problems? Will they be ICD9 diagnoses? Are there certain problems (HIV, behavioral health diagnoses) you won't include? Can the patient enter their problems?

- ✔ **Assessments and histories:** Medical, surgical, and family histories. Allow patients to update?

- ✔ **Visit summary:** Clinic visit, Emergency Department discharge summary, or discharge summary from hospital?

- ✔ **Education materials:** Will you use third-party content or links to other sites? Remember if you supply the link, you're responsible for the quality of the content.

- ✔ **Reminders:** Preventive health (mammogram, immunizations) and disease/medication–specific (regular lab tests for medications) alerts.

You don't have to provide electronic access to every note you make about a patient. Your EHR system may not allow you to do so. For example, you can use the EHR's security features to create a level of access that allows patients to see all the information they need to manage their self-care but doesn't let them see their entire legal medical record.

Ask your vendor what communication features the EHR offers. You can likely choose what you want, or even decide to add more features later.

Sharing test results

Communicating test results can be a shaky proposition because of the sensitivity of the tests' nature and the results. Some practices permit front office staff to communicate normal test results to the patient via e-mail or message. If your practice allows this, remember that normal ranges vary for certain tests based upon the patient. A lab sending a result indicating the value is "normal" doesn't mean the physician may not need to be notified of the result and follow-up with the patient.

Often, test results are sensitive in nature and, frankly, best reported in person, so your practice may want to consider developing a policy for communicating test results to patients. You can set up a series of if-then statements to direct employees on how to report all kinds of test information. For example, if a patient is tested for a sexually transmitted disease, results are always communicated in person. Or, if a routine Pap test is negative for abnormalities, the patient may be notified via secure e-mail. Use your judgment and experience to help keep your test result communications appropriate.

Educating patients about accessing information

Your communication efforts don't mean much if the patients don't know they can access their health records and communicate with your practice online. Therefore, a vital component of this new patient-centered communication system is helping patients understand how they can access their PHI and use the EHR tools you designate to communicate with physicians and practice staff members. You can

- ✔ Dedicate some space on your practice's Web site to discussing communication options.

- ✔ Provide patients with examples of the "best" reasons for an e-visit.

- ✔ Make sure that all your staff appropriately encourage/educate patients about their communication options.

- ✔ Create materials, such as flyers, handouts, and signs, to remind patients about such services as secure messaging, e-visits, and patient portals.

- ✔ Be clear and describe the process for how patients can start using e-visits and secure messaging. Tell patients they can

    - • Talk with staff and their doctor about secure messaging.

    - • Review the guidelines and privacy and security measures.

    - • Log in from home and start communicating.

One of the simplest ways you can educate patients about their communication options is to use the face time you already have. When you're in front of the computer with the patient for the first time, use that as an opportunity to discuss how the patient can access the same information that you do. Show them what their health records look like onscreen and walk them through the process of logging on and accessing their PHI. If you plan to offer e-mail or messaging functions, you (or another staff member) can show them how to check their inbox or IM page to send and receive communications from your practice.

Host a few communication seminars for your patients at various times, so you can focus 100 percent on showing them how to access their information and use the new e-mail and IM features. To increase patient attendance, put out some food, offer door prizes, and make it fun.

You can also educate patients about their communication options in other ways. Create some educational materials to pass out at each patient visit, include the information on your Web site, offer some in-person or Web-based seminars, or send out information with each bill to inform patients of their access rights and capabilities. Regardless of how you educate patients, be proactive and address common concerns, such as privacy and finances. You'll have a tech-savvy patient population in no time!

E-Mailing Your Patients

E-mail, often called secure messaging within the EHR, is the first big communications tool you should consider using in conjunction with your practice's new EHR. It's one of the most efficient and cost-conscious ways to communicate information about everything from appointment reminders and payment schedules to simple lab results or prescription questions. If your patients can type — even those that fall in the "hunt and peck" category — they're good candidates for e-mail!

If the vendor offers secure messaging capability with the EHR, find out what the security features are and whether (and how) the system creates an audit trail for e-mails, updates, and backups to the server that holds the e-mail data.

Enjoying messaging benefits

Communicating with patients via e-mail has its advantages, and you should consider those during your decision-making process. You and your staff can use e-mail to correspond with patients to

- ✔ Engage your patients more. They want to connect with you!
- ✔ Reduce unnecessary visits to the office so that you can focus on the patients who need to visit.
- ✔ Increase patient satisfaction. E-mail can be more convenient for the patient.
- ✔ Provide immediate care for a patient who otherwise might not get in the office for a week or longer.
- ✔ Handle administrative and scheduling questions through secure messaging.

Of course, there's the ever-present topic of cost savings. Although you might spend extra cash up front, purchasing an EHR with e-mail functionality will save you money in the long term because you can reduce the number of office visits, ER visits, and hospitalizations by providing faster, more efficient care via the technology.

Secure messaging through the EHR, as cheap and efficient as it is, can never replace a patient's face time with a physician. Use caution when you are setting up the parameters for what you will and will not discuss with a patient via e-mail. Save the in-depth discussions for an office visit and reserve your e-mail time for quick queries, reporting test results, setting appointment reminders, and other day-to-day office functions and concerns.

Overcoming obstacles

Secure messaging isn't a panacea for all your patient communication woes and needs. You can bet there will be challenges and maybe even a little push-back from patients who aren't very tech-savvy or employees who might feel that the practice's personal touch is lost on a computer screen.

The obvious obstacle for patient e-mail is privacy and security. Patients will be concerned about what is shared via the EHR. You and your staff need to discuss what measures are in place to ensure that their personal information is safe. If you decided to use the messaging features at the time of implementation, you can include this information on your initial patient education information about privacy and security (see Chapter 10). If you opt for the e-mail features later, you can always create a separate brochure. Additionally, offer some privacy and safety reassurance during patient visits.

You may view finance as a potential obstacle as well, primarily in terms of payment and reimbursement. You probably want to know whether you'll be paid for offering e-mail capability. Look into these options:

✔ Large insurers, such as Blue Cross, Aetna, and Cigna are reimbursing physicians for online visits. Visit `www.bcbsnc.com/content/providers/evisit.htm` for more information.

✔ Some malpractice carriers are reducing premiums for practices that use e-visits. Contact your carrier to find out whether you qualify.

✔ Code for the e-visit in your EHR using CPT code 99444. The Level I reimbursement code for online evaluation and management services provided by a physician can only be used with an established patient once every seven days.

Worrying that you and your staff will have to spend all day answering patient e-mails and have less time to spend helping people in person is understandable. Perhaps you worry that you'll just have to manage more patients. Anecdotal interviews and studies have found that practices become more efficient with the use of secure messaging and e-visits. Like many new workflows you'll experience with EHR, e-visits are also about sharing the workload. Front office staff and nurses can manage some messaging and route only the appropriate clinical messages to the physicians. Use your EHR-related staff meetings to determine what kind of e-mail workflow is most efficient for your practice.

Using messaging to its full potential

As soon as you decide to board the e-mail train, you can determine how, exactly, you want to use messaging to help your patients manage their care. Your level of dependence on this type of communication is up to both you and your patient. After all, you don't want to use e-mail communication with someone who doesn't like using a computer or checks his or her inbox on a limited basis.

When broaching the subject of e-mail with patients, ask whether they're interested in communicating with you electronically and provide them a list of topics covering what you might communicate. Allow patients to choose what topics they would like you to communicate via e-mail so that you share only the information they want and will use in their self-care management.

Here are some common uses for patient e-mail:

- ✔ Prescription renewals
- ✔ Answering questions
- ✔ Communicating with office staff about co-pays and health insurance
- ✔ Scheduling and rescheduling of appointments
- ✔ Answering colleague or specialist questions about problems
- ✔ Notifying patient population about additional services or classes. Example: *Remember that Thursday night we do diabetes education. Join us!*
- ✔ Reinforcing a treatment plan

Ask your patients what they would like to see you address via e-mail. Remember they are your consumers. Therefore, rely on them to tell you what their e-needs are.

When you work to establish the parameters of your e-mail communications plan, some best practices can help you use patient e-mail appropriately and to its fullest potential:

- ✔ **Set guidelines for your staff and your patients, and manage everyone's expectations upfront.** Communicate any fees that the patient might be responsible for — the costs for the practice and patient aren't high, but communicate them clearly. Some practices find it most useful to charge patients for an e-mail package as an extra service to cover costs.

- ✔ **Keep e-mails professional.** Don't use patient e-mail to forward your favorite joke of the day or use off-color language with patients. Be clear with your language — no abbreviations and acronyms. Although e-mail is known for its brevity, take the time and space to explain terms and common physician lingo so patients are not confused.

Make sure that your directives and instructions are clear and to the point. For example, be sure that patients know when an e-visit is not appropriate and they need to come into the office. Both patients and office staff should know what conditions should be discussed and assessed in person. E-visits and secure messaging are not great tools for managing someone's chest pain. By setting some parameters about what language is appropriate to use, you can keep the quality of the care you deliver at the high level your patients expect and deserve.

Visit `www.transformed.com/e-Visits/e-Visits_Scherger.cfm` for more information about patient e-mail best practices and risk management.

Introducing Patient Portals and PHRs

There is more to life than e-mail, and much of it exists on the Web in living color. You can use tools like patient portals and personal health records (PHRs) to engage your patient population even more fully in their self-care management. These features can include all the information you want and only the tools that apply to your patients' needs.

Be sure your vendor offers secure messaging, lab communication features, immunization reports, scheduling features, educational materials, fillable and printable forms, and prescription functions for your patient portal. For portals and PHRs, find out whether your vendor provides editing functions for providers and multiple language options.

Patient portals

A *patient portal* is a secure online application that lets you communicate with patients any time, day or night. Many EHRs offer a Web-based patient portal application that links to your EHR server, so patients can be active participants in the management of their healthcare.

A common feature of a patient portal is secure messaging (see the "E-Mailing Your Patient" section earlier in this chapter). Additionally, most portals allow patients to perform such tasks as posting new health developments or asking questions of their providers. Most portals allow patients to fill out forms online prior to an office or hospital visit, request prescription refills, view and print their medical records, confirm billing statements and arrange for online payments, view lab results or diagnostic images, and schedule or change appointments.

Figure 15-1 shows a patient portal.

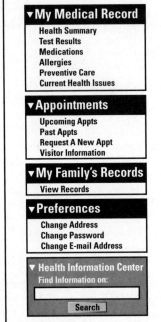

My Medical Record

Health Summary
Test Results
Medications
Allergies
Preventive Care
Current Health Issues

Appointments

Upcoming Appts
Past Appts
Request A New Appt
Visitor Information

My Family's Records

View Records

Preferences

Change Address
Change Password
Change E-mail Address

Health Information Center
Find Information on:

[Search]

Past Appointments

Click on a row to see your test results

Date/Time	Visit With	Department
Wednesday 10/17/2010	Your Physician	Internal Medicine
Monday 10/15/2010	Your Physician	Dermatology
Monday 08/20/2010	Your Physician	Internal Medicine
Thursday 07/20/2010	Your Physician	Internal Medicine

Click on a past appointment to view visit details of that appointment.

My Family's Records

Access another account

The MyChart Caregiver service has been granted for the family members listed below. Click a name to access that family member's MyChart account.

Patient	Access Until	Account Status
John Doe	09/17/2018	Active
Jane Doe		Inactive
Jay Random	02/10/2019	Active

The MyChart Caregiver service allows you to view family members' records. When clicking on a particular name, you will access that family member's MyChart account.

Figure 15-1:
A patient portal.

We mention in Chapter 2 that a patient portal goes a long way toward Meaningful Use (and the resulting incentive money). You can set up the portal to reflect aspects of Meaningful Use that you want to ensure your practice can prove. Most portals let practices decide what functions to use and what information to share, but it's not as easy as turning on the feature and just letting patients start using the portal. As an organization, you'll have to decide what makes sense for you. Remember that you don't have to turn everything on all at one time.

For more info about patient portals, see www.patientportalguru.com.

You can help patients acclimate to their new virtual view of the healthcare world by offering assistance in the form of handouts, special workshops, or hands-on demonstrations as time allows. You can also ease their tech fears by working with the vendor to make sure that online forms look like your practice's traditional paper forms.

What to ask your vendor about patient portals

You can make sure you are getting the most bang for your EHR buck by asking your vendor some questions about the portal capabilities your EHR offers. Be sure to ask about the following:

Messaging: How does the messaging capability work? Are messages saved in the EHR? How? Are messages part of the patient's chart? How do I know if the patient has read my message? What are the messaging security features?

Lab results: How do patients get their results? Can I set up parameters for the results that are relayed online? How does the portal handle abnormal results? How do patients communicate questions about lab results? Can patients find links to more information? Can patients print test results?

CCDs and CCRs: Does your product support the import and export of Continuity of Care Documents (CCDs) and/or Continuity of Care Records (CCR) from patients or other care sites, such as clinics or hospitals? Are problem lists, medication lists, allergy lists, and test results included? What isn't included?

Reimbursements: Can you support reimbursement for e-visits through the portal? Is the portal capable of processing credit card payments?

E-visits: How does the portal route e-visit requests? Can the portal customize patient questionnaires? Can a provider set parameters for e-visit frequency? How does the portal allow a provider to comply with laws or regulations concerning visits?

Billing: How do you support billing services through your portal? Can patients pay their bills online? Are there extra costs or license fees when using the billing features? Can patients obtain e-statements? Can they opt out of paper statements?

Caregivers: How do you support proxy access for parents or caregivers? Can the portal filter features based on who (if not the patient) is viewing the record? How can I control proxy access to records? Can patients determine what others can and cannot see on their record? Can I audit proxy access?

Site administration: Who handles the administration of the site and its use? How do patients reset login and password information? Can we outsource our help desk? Do you offer Web-based administrative tools? What about admin security? Can we set up an admin audit trail? Is there a way to track patient calls?

E-prescribing: Can you support prescription management, including requests and integration with pharmacies? What tools are available to help us manage patient prescription messages? How does the portal work with pharmacy directories?

Information management: How can the practices decide what information to share with the patient? How do patients view the portal? Can patients print or export their information? Does the portal link to any registries? What about HIE, hospitals, and other clinics?

Personal health records

Personal health records (PHRs) are another great way to open the lines of communication with your patients. Figure 15-2 shows a personal health record.

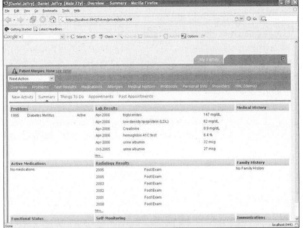

Figure 15-2:
Offer your patients access to their personal health record.

A PHR is a tool that operates independently of your practice's EHR; however, it can work with your EHR. Owned and managed by the patient, the PHR can include any information from a clinical setting that the patient wants in the record. Ideally, a PHR allows patients to collect, store, manage, and share their personal health information with physicians, specialists, and designated caregivers while retaining its portability. Whether a patient has new insurance, switches physicians, or changes jobs, his or her PHR information should remain the same and offer the same accessibility.

PHRs can help patients manage the following types of information:

✔ Demographic information

✔ Problem list and diagnoses list

✔ Medication list

✔ Allergies

✔ Diagnostic test results

✔ Procedures and surgeries

✔ Doctor/hospital visit history

✔ Family medical history

✔ Remote monitoring data

✔ Immunization history

Several good Web sites provide patients details about selecting a PHR. Some PHRs are usually offered through employers and health plans, and others are available for purchase or offered through health systems. Try www.medicare.gov/navigation/manage-your-health/personal-health-records/learn-more-phr.aspx and www.nlm.nih.gov/medlineplus/personalhealthrecords.html.

Patient action is another key element of a PHR. Your patients should not only view information but also use tools that help them manage their care. The PHR should offer data about claims, potential medication interactions or allergies, billing action items, and other health information. Hopefully, your patient's PHR will offer such functions as secure messaging, data personalization, and document management.

A study conducted by the Center for Information Technology Leadership projected that interoperable PHRs can save the U.S. healthcare industry $19 billion annually.

A patient portal and PHR may appear the same on the surface, but some characteristics separate the two. Table 15-2 outlines the differences.

Table 15-2	Patient Portals versus PHRs
Patient Portal	**PHR**
An extension of the EHR and the practice/hospital	Separate, independent tool/software
Most information and interaction is driven by the practice	Owned and managed by the patient
Generally tied to one practice or health system	Ability to include information from all clinical settings
Most information is codified and structured (lab results, medication lists)	Ability to capture both structured and free text information — free text information is managed by the patient
Limited ability for patient-entered data	Allows for patient-entered data
Many import and export summary care record using the Continuity of Care Document (CCD) or Continuity of Care Record (CCR) standards for problems, medications, allergies, and lab results	Can export and import summary care records using the Continuity of Care Document (CCD) or Continuity of Care Record (CCR) standards for the majority of data stored in the PHR
Used primarily for viewing of health information by patients	Used primarily for management of health information by patients

PHRs are on the rise. Check out these PHR stats cited in "The Integrated Personal Health Record and the Involved Consumer," a white paper by WebMD Health Services:

- ✔ In 2008, 7.3 million U.S. adults used an online personal health record and 72.5 million U.S. adults reported interest in using an online PHR. (Source: "Cybercitizen Health v8.0," Manhattan Research, 2009.)

- ✔ Fifty-seven percent of consumers surveyed want a secure Internet site to access medical records, schedule office visits, refill prescriptions, and pay medical bills. (Source: "Survey of Health Care Consumers," Deloitte Center for Health Solutions, 2009.)

- ✔ Fifty-five percent of consumers surveyed want to use e-mail to exchange health information with doctors. (Source: "Survey of Health Care Consumers," Deloitte Center for Health Solutions, 2009.)

- ✔ Seventy-nine percent of consumers surveyed believe using an online PHR would provide major benefits in managing their health and healthcare services. (Source: "Connecting for Health," Markle Foundation, 2008.)

- ✔ Sixty-five percent of consumers surveyed are interested in home monitoring devices that enable them to check their condition and send the results to their doctor. (Source: "Survey of Health Care Consumers: Key Findings, Strategic Implication," Deloitte Center for Health Solutions, 2009.)

Obviously, patient interest in PHRs is high, and the potential for greater efficiency, lower costs, and — most importantly — a more engaged patient population is great. Pretty good reasons to help your patients set up their own PHRs and then integrate them with your EHR.

Chapter 16

Improving and Tweaking the System

Someone once said that the only constant is change. It can be true in life and very true with your EHR. Though your new EHR isn't necessarily a living, breathing entity, it's managed by living, breathing people — all of whom are capable of affecting how the technology works and changes.

As time goes on, your system needs to change with your practice. Maybe you no longer need some of your EHR's features, or perhaps you need to add functionality. You might need to improve your reporting capabilities or work to meet new, updated Meaningful Use guidelines (and there will be some, we promise). No matter what kind of change comes your way, you need to be ready to roll with it and improve your systems to meet your practice's ever-changing needs.

Traveling the Long Road to Get It Right

Life is all about the journey, and your EHR is, too. While familiarizing yourself with what the system offers and what you can accomplish when you use it, you'll start to make some connections between your goals and your use of the EHR. What you find might surprise you. You may find that you don't really use as many of the bells and whistles as you thought, or that you need some features less regularly than you thought. The reality is that you'll most likely take advantage of less than 50 percent of your EHR capabilities and functions.

Set yourself up for a reality check. There's nothing wrong with including all the functional tools that your heart desires in your initial EHR package — just know that your needs change and so will your EHR over time.

Realize that implementation and go-live are merely the beginning stages of your new life with the EHR. There will be a lot more to think about after all the e-dust settles, and it's a good idea to start crafting a plan now for life after go-live. While all your questions and ideas are fresh in your head, think about how you want to handle post–go-live training and system optimization.

Step one of creating this plan is to speak with your vendor about how best to maintain an ongoing relationship with your rep and any other inside contacts (such as vendor-based technical support staff) you utilize. Some of your ongoing vendor relationship may be outlined in your contract, but think about what you might need from your rep that isn't spelled out in ink.

Most reps want to keep your business, so they're often willing to provide you with support services that aren't noted in the contract. It never hurts to ask!

Regardless of how you want to use the EHR in the coming months and years, know that there will likely never be an "A-ha!" moment when everything clicks and works perfectly. Your practice is constantly changing, and you will want to use your EHR in ways that reflect that change. When you discover new needs, you have an opportunity to address them using the powerful tools of your EHR. The long road to EHR nirvana is quite a journey, so buckle up and get ready for the ride.

Creating a Long-Term Support Strategy

Having a support strategy is vital to the longevity and health of your EHR because, we hope, you're going to be together for a very long time. Therefore, it's important that you not only think about the support that you need right away and in the coming months, but in the long term, too.

Think about what resources you will need to get the support you want. You can start by answering these questions:

- ✔ Is someone in-house, the vendor, or an outside entity going to maintain the system?

- ✔ Can you make changes to the system without the vendor's help?

- ✔ How will you monitor the EHR to know when it needs updating or fixing, and when you might need to rethink whether it's meeting your needs?

- ✔ How much ongoing training do you want? Will you need training for each major upgrade or update?

- ✔ How do you want to handle the training of new employees?

✔ How can you offer training and ongoing education without completely disrupting your workflows?

✔ What should your long-term evaluative systems look like? What kind of reports and audits should you take part in? Will it serve your needs to have both objective and subjective data?

Choosing a vendor support model

One important source of support is your vendor. He will probably offer several different long-term support options, similar to your go-live support:

✔ **Remote support:** All support is provided online and via phone.

✔ **Onsite support:** The vendor support rep visits your office on a regular basis to offer support and assistance. This may not be practical (too many cooks in the kitchen) or necessary.

✔ **A combination of the two:** Onsite dedicated support is offered to help with workflows and using the system as designed. A level of remote support is used to troubleshoot technical issues.

When you determine what support level you need, you can hammer out the logistics with the vendor rep and document the person each employee and workstation should call for support.

Supporting yourself

In addition to the vendor, you are a great source of support. The more that you and your staff can do in the system, the better off you will be. Rather than paying someone to tweak your EHR or waiting to get an update from the vendor, you can learn to make changes yourself when you need them. Many vendors offer specific training classes to help you become efficient in building and designing your EHR.

Here are some things you can do to support yourself:

✔ **Vendor training:** Many vendors provide a formal training program for their clients, which is a great way to become more self-sufficient as a trainer or builder in the EHR. Generally, classes are held at the vendor's headquarters and you dedicate two to three weeks to become "certified" in the EHR.

✔ **Web site:** Your vendor may have a Web site where you can share materials with other practices. For example, you can find physician notes and quality reports that you can tweak for your office.

- ✔ **Conferences:** Typically, vendors host annual conferences for their clients. This is a great opportunity to discover what other practices are doing and what new features the vendor is rolling out. (Before you know it, you might even be presenting at the next conference.) You also make great contacts with other practices and can share information regularly.

- ✔ **Local groups:** Work with other practices in your area. Many times the best sources of information are the clinicians who are using an EHR daily.

- ✔ **RECs:** Your Regional Extension Center can provide valuable information about the use and optimization of different EHRs. The center can also connect you with other local practices and support resources.

Using support tools

You can create a whole library of support tools to make available to your practice's employees so they can have the resources they need to succeed with the EHR. There is so much great, free information about EHRs available on the Web and from outside resources, you'd be hard pressed not to find something useful on how to use them and how to make the most of your experience with them.

While you familiarize yourself with the system, turn your notes into quick, easy-to-read tip sheets that others in the office can use. Keep your support materials concise and focused on specific features. Provide screenshots and step-by-step instructions for your staff and colleagues. You can also use a simple, handheld video camera to create your own mini podcasts or video tutorials to use during the training of new hires and retraining for existing employees.

The Web has a slew of EHR-related Web sites, many of which offer free, short instructional videos.

Make use of any outside help you can find. Think about what outside resources you can use to help your staff continue their EHR training and retraining, and optimize their experience with the system. We outline several resources in Chapter 3.

Your support system really does have to be a priority if you want to keep using the EHR into your practice's golden years. Therefore, use people invested in your success, both in and out of the clinical setting, to ensure that your EHR lasts for years to come and that you get the most out of not only your financial investment, but your investments of time and talent, too.

Reporting: Learning from What You Do Every Day

A vital part of your long-term EHR strategy is to make use of the reports you create every day. You may have been conducting quality reporting before, but perhaps not as efficiently as you sorted through charts to find and measure specific clinical information. Because your EHR software can create reports on just about every aspect of how you use the system, you can have a full record of how you conduct the practice's business each day. And the best part of having those reports is that you can chart and track how you are using the EHR and how it's serving your needs.

The patterns of data that you use to note trends in patient care and indicate ways to improve how you deliver that care can change over time as you tweak your system and resulting workflows. Consider the following while you tweak your reporting process:

- ✔ What measures you need to review on a regular basis
- ✔ Who can run and review reports
- ✔ How you will communicate the information to your staff and colleagues
- ✔ How the information will help you change your care delivery
- ✔ Whether the data fields are consistently filled out in the EHR so that the reports are accurate and complete
- ✔ How easy it is to customize or create new reports

Much of your data can be used to help you prove that you're using — or not using — the EHR in a meaningful way that improves quality.

Your office team plays an integral role in deciding how you want to set up quality reporting. Ask for their input on what patient information is most vital to quality reporting and have them assist in data collection in a way that complements how the functions of their roles.

Share your quality reports with staff at regular intervals so you can amend workflows and note both large- and small-scale changes in your processes and workflows. Transparency with your staff, and even your patients, will help everyone improve.

Your reporting may not pay big dividends until a few months after you begin to use the EHR. Trends don't show immediately, so have some realistic expectations about what your reporting demonstrates. You can run reports about prescription management, billing, incentives, reimbursements, and just about anything else you can think of. Remember that many EHRs either include or connect to a quality reporting tool that you can customize to fit your needs, which beats memorizing and keeping track of such rules on an ongoing basis, and it is set up to update with the latest new information. You can access clinical guidelines, protocols, pay-for-performance initiatives, and formulary and Meaningful Use requirements. See whether your vendor posts materials from clients on its Web site and then take advantage of what other practices successfully have done before you.

You can use your EHR's quality reporting tools to access information about drug interactions and allergies, fulfill payment criteria, flag and amend possible billing errors, chart your participation in incentive programs, monitor reimbursement quality and frequency, and interact with and respond to federal mandates and programs.

Figure 16-1 shows an example of an EHR reporting tool.

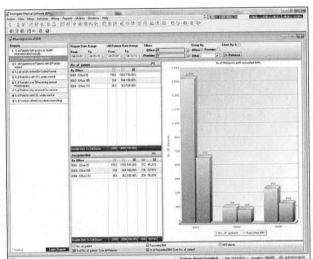

Figure 16-1:
EHR
reporting
tool.

Getting Help When You Need It

Something isn't working correctly with your EHR. Do you try to fix it in-house (risking an even greater problem down the road), do you call an outside IT specialist, or do you touch base with your vendor rep to see what help he or she can offer (if you don't already have a support plan with the vendor)?

Working with your vendor rep

When you need some help with your system, your first call should be to the vendor rep to report your problem and see what, if any, solutions, she can offer you as part of your existing support package. Many of your ongoing support issues concerning tweaking and improving your system will be supported by the vendor per the terms of your contract. For support that isn't spelled out in your contract, ask your rep.

Your vendor rep has likely seen all possible problems that could pop up with your system and can serve as a helpful resource. If the problem is more of a technical issue, then try to drill down the parameters of what is not working before you contact the rep. That way, you won't waste a lot of vendor support time attempting to diagnose the problem. Obviously, this isn't always feasible (sometimes you simply won't know what is wrong), but alerting the rep that your problem lies with a specific part of the system or how you use it streamlines your support time. The problem could be one of the following:

✔ **System:** Many EHRs offer online support to report problems or bugs by setting up a help desk (see Figure 16-2), which is an online form you can fill out and send to the vendor with the click of a button. You will also have a (hopefully) 24/7 help line that you can call. Alternately, if you think your rep will get the problem fixed faster, keep him or her on speed dial.

The caveat with vendor support issues is that the responsibility to follow up is on you. Perhaps the vendor doesn't call you back or fixes the problem without telling you. Always schedule time to check in and make sure the work is done to your satisfaction.

✔ **Interface:** The big question here is who owns the problem. Interface issues can be tricky. Your practice didn't create the interface, but there is a chance that the vendor used a third party to create it. To find out whose problem it really is, first consult your contract (and possibly your legal counsel) and then move forward with asking your vendor whom to ask for assistance.

✔ **Network:** This will probably be an issue that your internal IT folks or vendor IT technicians can fix. One of the biggest networking challenges is speed, and the problem likely boils down to a connectivity issue or security breach.

✔ **Workflow:** How you use the EHR in the practice is often more of a people issue than a technology issue. However, you can work with your vendor rep to brainstorm workflow solutions and potentially add different features to your EHR that will support what you want to accomplish.

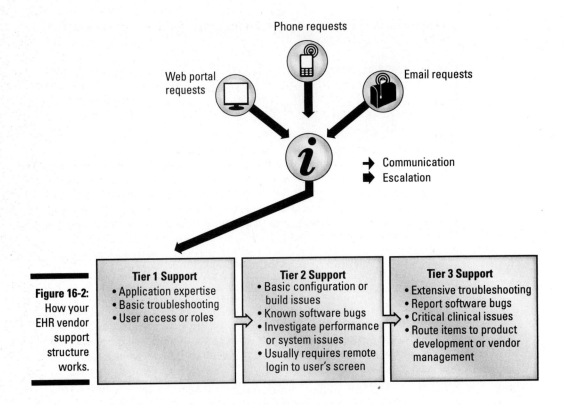

Figure 16-2:
How your
EHR vendor
support
structure
works.

Finding help outside the office

Other helpful resources are available to you outside of what your vendor can
provide. Additional help is available from Regional Extension Centers (RECs),
other health systems, and professional organizations. See Chapter 3 for help
finding your local Regional Extension Center.

Regional Extension Centers provide a range of services that you might get
free or for a few thousand dollars, depending on whether you qualify as a
priority provider and how services are packaged. Some of the post–go-live
services the REC might offer include

✔ Community forums to learn about local best practices

✔ Consulting services to improve your use of the EHR

✔ Loan programs for new hardware, software, or support services

✔ Interface development for labs, radiology sites, or hospitals

✔ Reporting support for immunization registries or national organizations

You can also look to health systems or hospitals for more assistance. They can help you with the following:

- **Vendor management:** If the hospital is using the same vendor, it can leverage its size and relationship to manage the vendor to set and maintain stringent performance benchmarks for both the technology and professional services, such as project management, system configuration, and training.

- **Facilities and ongoing training:** Many hospitals offer a place where you can look at the system and figure out what works best for your practice when you are thinking about adding features down the road. Hospitals and health systems often set up nice training programs — with a training room — to make sure that their providers have a good environment for training. They often set up training "test beds" where fake patients are set up so that you can go through more realistic training, too.

- **Interface maintenance:** Hospitals and health systems usually have IT departments that are dedicated to working with vendors to ensure that the interfaces are developed to meet requirements. When you need to update existing (or add new) interfaces, the hospital might be able to support you in that work.

- **Ongoing customer support:** If you implement an EHR offered by your local hospital, you're its EHR customer. In other words, a person answers when you call the support line. Your hospital wants your business, so it wants to provide you with good customer support.

Professional societies and organizations exist to support and help you. Find out about them in Chapter 3.

Additionally, remember the quality organizations while you continue to tweak how you use the EHR system, including the AHRQ, AQA, PCPI, AHQA, NCQA, NGC, and NQF. If you can't remember what all of those letters stand for, the appendix offers definitions of these acronyms.

Deciding to switch vendors

If your vendor rep no longer supports your product or goes out of business, consider switching providers. However, the search process and the reimplementation process can be long and arduous. Some estimates report that it can cost between $30,000 and $50,000 per provider to upgrade to a different system, so it obviously makes sense to tread lightly around the issue of vendor switching. If you opt to move on with another vendor, you'll need to account for how it affects your bottom line, your staff, your processes, and your workflows. You will likely have to dance around some of the same issues here that you did with the original EHR implementation. So exhaust all your options before switching your vendor.

Installing Fixes and Upgrades from the Vendor

Fixes and upgrades allow your system to run at optimal efficiency and provide you with the most recent resources and tools to help you improve your practice's processes and workflows.

But you can't get that new functionality without going through the training process. Though it won't be on the same scale as your initial training and implementation, count on spending some time training after you install upgrades to your system, even if that means you just take five minutes to address the change during a staff meeting. If not everyone knows about an update, then he or she certainly can't use the new feature.

When you're trying to determine what fixes and upgrades to add to your system, think of a big buffet with several interesting choices. If you choose everything, you'll be sick. You need to pick the fixes or upgrades that offer you the most functionality without overloading you and your employees. Here are some of the elements of the EHR you can choose to upgrade or change:

- ✔ Hosting model (ASP or local)
- ✔ Practice management software
- ✔ Template changes
- ✔ Adding or removing buttons and forms
- ✔ Changing reminders
- ✔ Changing what you can and cannot print
- ✔ Entry sorting
- ✔ Reporting features
- ✔ Case sorting
- ✔ Communication features

The vendor will update its system regularly but depending on the vendor, this might mean a small update every other month or a very large update every year. Talk with your vendor early so that you fully understand the process and can set expectations with your staff. The vendor will also supply you with documents that describe any updates or fixes to its software. You and your staff will need to decide what features to implement.

When you decide on what you want to fix or update, think about how the change will affect the clinical setting. You can determine the "real" cost of any major upgrades or fixes by working with employees to figure out who is affected and how. Table 16-1 lists how potential upgrades or fixes might affect some of your practice's existing roles and workflows.

Table 16-1	The Impact of Fixes and Upgrades
Role	*Impact*
EHR Champion or Primary Decision Maker	Reviews potential upgrades; manages decision-making process; reports to other stakeholders
EHR Transition Team	Takes time away from everyday roles to assist with decision making
Front Office	May have to slow patient flow to accommodate upgrade and potentially new or amended workflows
Nursing Staff	May have to participate in extended training; expect a period of slowed workflows and processes
Physician	Possible primary decision maker; serves as champion for upgrade changes
Billing Staff	Potential workflow changes; possible slowed billing cycle during upgrade installation and training
Patients	Could experience slower wait times and difficulty getting an appointment due to temporary reduction in patient flow

Your vendor rep is an excellent resource for determining what fixes and upgrades your practice needs to add to your existing EHR. They can advise you on the potential effects an upgrade will have on staff, how the upgrade or fix is going to be installed or configured (sometimes a new build is required), and what kind of interface or screen changes you'll see.

Deciding When and Why to Add More Functionality

You may have taken the "dip your toes in the pool" approach to implementing your EHR and only added the basic features and functions you thought your practice needed to succeed. Now that you're an old hand at this whole EHR thing, you might want to consider adding more functionality to your system.

There are as many ways to advance the use of your EHR as there are stars in the sky, but the following sections cover two big ones: physician remote access and patient remote monitoring.

Adding remote access

Getting rid of that paper chart safety net means that physicians can no longer grab a chart and make notes or update information during rounds or offsite activities. Adding remote access increases your efficiency and provides increased productivity. Perhaps you want to see your schedule for later in the day while you're rounding in the hospital. Maybe you want home access so you can update charts in your pajamas. Now when you're on call, you can review a patient's key clinical information before you tell them to go to the emergency room or not. Depending on your vendor, a smartphone app may exist for accessing patient charts.

You always have security and privacy concerns when accessing patient records remotely. Check with your vendor rep to make sure that you're getting the functionality you want with the security you and your patients demand. Check out Chapter 10 for more information about maintaining your EHR's security features away from the clinical setting.

Giving patients remote access

Patient remote monitoring is a feature you might want to install if your patients want to share their home monitoring info (blood pressure, blood glucose readings) with you. Patients can use digitally connected medical diagnostic devices to report data to their doctors from the comfort of their home.

Remote access is an especially functional addition to your EHR for several reasons, the biggest of which is that it allows you to keep track of vital data without dragging patients into the office on a regular basis or requiring them to keep cumbersome paper records of their numbers. For example, a patient can use a portable electrocardiogram (ECG) to monitor his heart rate throughout the day. The ECG automatically reports this data to the EHR site, and the patient record populates. Then when the physician checks the numbers that evening in his or her living room, the data is there. And no one had to leave home.

You can use remote monitoring to manage just about any type of regularly reported self-care. You could provide remote monitoring for the purposes of communicating physiologic measurements (weight, blood pressure, heart rate and rhythm, pulse oximetry, glucose), diagnostic measurements (transthoracic impedance), device information (medication pumps, electronic pillboxes, infusion devices, ADL biosensors, pedometers), and daily measurements (sleep actigraphy), to name a few.

Consider how to implement the workflows for remote patient monitoring. MDs don't always want to see daily measurements or be responsible (or liable) for monitoring data daily. Other clinical staff members are usually charged with managing this kind of information on a day-to-day level. Typically, that responsibility falls to the nursing staff.

Some reports indicate that using patient remote monitoring can reduce hospitalizations by up to 50 percent.

Remote monitoring is fairly intuitive. When a patient's numbers are off-kilter, an instant notification can be sent to the monitoring party (often nurses). This allows the staff to follow up and address the patient's problem immediately. Without remote monitoring, patient (especially the homebound with chronic diseases) problems can go unnoticed for several days. Patients don't always notice or report minor changes in their conditions to doctors, and those changes often aren't discovered until a nurse makes a scheduled visit, which could be days after the patient develops the problem.

Some insurers and other healthcare payers don't always reimburse providers for remote monitoring services or devices. Check before you implement this feature.

Participating and Contributing to a Health Information Exchange

A major reason to tweak and update your system is so you can engage more actively in a *health information exchange,* or *HIE*. An HIE is healthcare information that is shared across organizations from varying hospital, community, or regional systems. An HIE allows you to share patient data with other hospital systems and share in continuity of care. HIE also allows you to communicate across system lines, maintain the integrity of patient information, and contribute information to public health entities. The more information you can supply to your local health department (and similar groups), the easier it is for them to chart the health of the population at large and prevent communicable diseases.

HIE is a part of Meaningful Use, especially in 2013 and 2015.

While you determine what kind of HIE-related functionality you want to add to your EHR, you should ask yourself some questions so that you create a system that's conducive to your level of HIE involvement:

✔ Does your health system's EHR connect to their hospitals? (This hospital may be connecting to the regional or state HIE.)

✔ Does your REC or EHR vendor include an HIE interface?

✔ What is the cost of integrating with your regional or state HIE? Potential HIE integration levels include

- *Separate portal:* You can log in and look up the patient again. This is not preferred because you'll rarely log in.

- *Interfaced:* You have a link to launch or view the data in the HIE application.

- *Integrated:* You can see HIE data within your EHR (within a tab or view of your EHR).

When you know the answers to these questions, you can work more closely with your vendor rep to determine how your EHR can help you harness the power of the HIE to report data that can help other practices and public health entities.

Finding HIE help

Several good HIE resources can help you navigate the often choppy waters of exchanging information. Regional health information organizations (RHIOs) and state-level organizations provide information exchange terms and requirements, and develop methods and standards for the exchange of health information. Here are a few resources we like:

HIELights: A monthly e-newsletter subscription focused on RHIO and HIE initiatives:

www.himss.org/ASP/topics_
     FocusDynamic.asp?faid=156

RHIO/HIE Industry References: A compendium of general HIE information and links to organizations that support the implementation of health information exchange entities:

www.himss.org/ASP/topics_
     FocusDynamic.asp?faid=142

RHIO/HIE Educational Tools: HIMSS educational references and resources:

www.himss.org/ASP/topics_
     FocusDynamic.asp?faid=141

eHealth Initiative (eHI): Not-for-profit organization whose mission is to drive the quality, safety, and efficiency of healthcare through information and information technology. The eHI Web site includes a map of HIE activity in the United States:

www.ehealthinitiative.org

Integrating the Health Enterprise (IHE): More than 200 member organizations (including professional and trade associations, vendors, researchers, and providers) focused on improving interoperability between health systems. IHE sponsors the Connectathon, where vendors utilize test systems and scripts to demonstrate interoperability:

www.ihe.net

NHINWatch: Updates and information on the Nationwide Health Information Network (NHIN) and HIE initiatives across the nation:

www.nhinwatch.com

This is just a small sampling of the wealth of HIE resources on the Web. So get your Google skills in shape, get on the Internet, and start finding some resources of your own! Your Regional Extension Center also knows about the HIE initiatives in your state, so contact it or your local hospital to learn about your options.

Take note if your EHR's decision support rules are not using the HIE data. If you see something in the HIE for a patient, you still need to practice good clinical care and get an accurate history from the patient as well as determine what needs to be documented within your EHR. The alerts and rules can only fire on data within your EHR, not the HIE. The HIE is a resource for you — an opportunity to view Emergency Room discharge summaries, other encounter notes, lab results, medications, and so on. So, use it as a reference.

Part V
The Part of Tens

The 5th Wave   By Rich Tennant

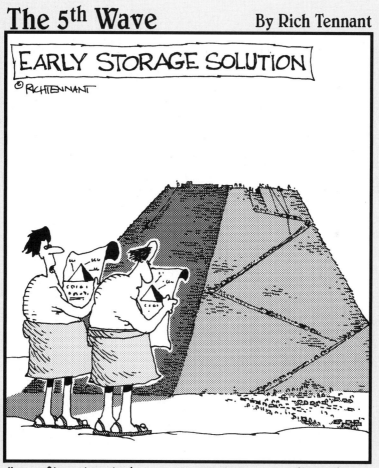

"Configuring it has been a little tougher than we thought."

In this part . . .

This part is full of quick, easy-to-pick-up information. Chapter 17 shines the spotlight on ten useful Web sites (although we calculate a gazillion EHR-related sites are out there). Chapter 18 troubleshoots what we think your top EHR problems might be. Chapter 19 asks, "So, what's your question?" and covers the top ten questions you need to ask and answer.

Chapter 17

Ten EHR-Related Web Sites

*W*hen you're in full-on EHR mode, the online world is where you find the great majority of your medical technology information. You can harness the power of the Internet to find just about anything you ever wanted to know about healthcare information technology and EHR in particular. An infinite number of individual vendor sites, health tech blogs, and metasites sponsored by the federal government and trade associations are dedicated to all things EHR. Here are a few of our favorites.

HIMSS.org

The Healthcare Information and Management Systems Society (HIMSS) is one of the preeminent organizations in all of health care. Its national organization and state chapters support clinical, IT, and administrative members with a wide variety of healthcare IT topics, including quality improvement, EHR adoption, and information integration. HIMSS has more than 23,000 members, and approximately 73 percent of them work in patient care delivery settings. To explore the site's EHR-specific content, click Electronic Health Record under the Topics section to find content on adoption, return on investment, EHR standards, tools, white papers, information on usability, case studies, and sample documents.

The HIMSS EHR Association is a trade organization of EHR companies; its Web site (www.HIMSSEHRA.org) discusses national EHR adoption issues and concerns and is a good place to find content about current news and initiatives. You can find information on the association's various workgroups, statements and positions, healthcare initiatives, and association partners. The site also showcases various quick start guides and case studies.

AmericanEHR.com

AmericanEHR Partners is a Web-based, vendor-neutral resource for EHR system selection and implementation developed by the American College of Physicians (ACP) and Cientis Technologies. This resource can help physicians as they face the intimidating task of selecting and implementing a system.

Participating professional societies include the following:

✔ American College of Physicians (ACP)

✔ American Academy of Allergy

✔ Asthma & Immunology (AAAAI)

✔ American College of Rheumatology (ACR)

✔ American Osteopathic Association of Medical Informatics (AOAMI)

✔ American Psychiatric Association, Infectious Diseases Society of America (IDSA)

✔ Renal Physicians Association (RPA)

✔ Society of General Internal Medicine (SGIM)

The site includes

✔ EHR readiness assessment tool to assess and gauge the effort and commitment required for EHR adoption

✔ EHR comparison engine and rating system, based on selected specialty and other search criteria, helps practices evaluate and compare products and user ratings

✔ Automated RFI to send to vendors

✔ Interactive physician community for sharing user experiences

✔ EHR blog with guest bloggers

✔ Biweekly EHR newsletter

✔ Specialty and sub-specialty society specific information and resources

✔ Educational resources and podcasts

✔ Links to participating RECs

CenterforHIT.org

The Center for Health Information Technology at the American Academy of Family Physicians site (www.centerforHIT.org) focuses on the process of seeking and selecting an EHR vendor. The site offers useful tools and forms and provides a step-by-step look at the EHR adoption process. Additionally, you can find tips, tutorials, discussion boards (for members), EHR reviews, resources for vendors, a readiness assessment tool, and the Find a Doctor Like Me in a Practice Like Mine tool. If you're an AAFP member, we definitely recommend this site.

HealthIT.HHS.gov

The Health Information Technology Web site (http://HealthIT.HHS.gov) of the Department of Health and Human Services hosts a great deal of information about the Health Information Technology for Economic and Clinical Health (HITECH) Act, which amends Title XXX of the Public Health Service Act by adding a number of funding opportunities for those seeking to advance health information technology. Check this site for Health Information Technology for Economic and Clinical Health (HITECH) Act programs; links to regional extension centers (as discussed in Chapter 3); regulations; blogs, twitter feeds; Meaningful Use information; and links to outreach, events, and other resources. Your Regional Extension Center (REC) can also be found on this site at http://healthit.hhs.gov/programs/REC.

HealthIT.AHRQ.gov

The plethora of links and information make the Agency for Healthcare Research and Quality site (www.ahrq.gov) a bit challenging to navigate but worth your time. You'll find a lot of information about all things healthcare IT, including a "knowledge library" boasting more than 6,000 resources as well as AHRQ-sponsored reports, links to EHR-related journal articles, an implementation checklist, e-prescribing info, health IT tools, and funding opportunities. The pics and bios of experts who contribute to the site put a face on the content, a nice touch. We recommend the Health IT Survey Compendium for publicly available EHR readiness assessments, patient surveys, and provider surveys.

HIStalk2.com

HIStalk, written by "Mr. HIStalk" (founder) and Inga (sidekick), who both have remained anonymous for 7 years, is a really interesting Web site with blogs, discussion forums, news, and other information focused on the health IT industry. HIStalk has gained a number of sponsors (without soliciting any), and is widely read, despite its anonymity.

HealthcareITnews.com

Published in partnership with the HIMSS, this is an all-healthcare IT, all the time news site with a wide-reaching variety of articles related to information technology that affect your day-to-day working environment. It has all the features of a typical industry-specific news site: links to the usual professional/social networking suspects (Twitter, LinkedIn), healthcare IT blogs and RSS feeds, job boards, and event listings. It also hosts or links to such resources as white papers, webinars, videos, and podcasts. One of the most useful features of the site is news organized by stakeholder interest. Under the Sections heading, you can see news grouped for hospitals and IDNs, physician practices and ambulatory care, payers, vendors, and international interests.

KLASResearch.com

We would be remiss to leave out the site where you can purchase the KLAS report. You can pay to get the detailed KLAS report, which summarizes objective and subjective reviews of almost all EHR vendor products using interviews from existing EHR clients, or just check out its Web site for plenty of accurate, free information. You can also search for a vendor on the home page to generate a basic vendor profile with contact information. The site offers a performance database, special reports, and advisory services along with custom research. A complimentary KLAS account is required to access much of the information.

EMRUpdate.com

This site boasts "unbiased independent EMR discussions," and delivers on that promise. In addition to offering several other useful tools for your vendor research phase, you'll find a plethora of EHR-related blogs, independent articles, discussion forums, and opinions of physicians and clinicians who have "been there, done that" in terms of vendor selection, go-live, and maintenance. The site also links to a wiki directory of vendors, suppliers, consultants, and training providers and a wiki of EHR terminology and basic facts. Be aware, though, that the site is ad-sponsored, so you have to look past a lot of junk.

You can use many great online tools to help guide your EHR vendor choice. We like www.ehrselector.com. There is a reasonable fee, but hey, your sanity is worth it.

EMRConsultant.com

This free Web site allows you to create a profile and match it to potential vendors that meet your specific selection criteria. You can receive up to five customized recommendations free. The interface is eye-catching, with the profile set up to look like a paper medical chart. Who says you can't have a little fun with a serious topic? The site also offers information on stimulus incentive programs that comply with the HITECH Act (hello, extra income). Additionally, you can find a great deal of EMR and EHR educational information, including a primer on the difference between the two. Check out the link to EHRTv.com, which showcases all sorts of video clips and interviews. Look closely for all the extra goodies the site offers; they're in a very small font at the bottom of the main page. Trust us — they're worth finding.

Chapter 18

Ten Problems (And Solutions) You'll Face

*W*e'd love to tell you that adopting, implementing, and maintaining your EHR will be perfect, seamless processes. And for the most part, they can be. The EHR isn't infallible and neither are we, which means that ultimately, you'll have problems. Think of this chapter as a little premarital counseling. This chapter details ten possible problems that you face as you research, select, and implement your new EHR.

Pinpointing Your Needs

You see other clinicians' EHRs and think, "Wow. That could be us." However, the truth is that those EHRs couldn't be you because each office, clinic, and hospital has very different EHR needs based on individual circumstances. You must examine your situation very carefully to determine what *you* need from EHR. The process of making that determination is complex because you must address several issues including, but not limited to

✔ What you want to change about your workflow and the opportunities for increased efficiency

✔ How each stakeholder group, from physicians to patients, needs to interact with the EHR information

✔ What financial improvements you hope to gain from EHR

✔ How you want patient involvement to improve

✔ What errors in charting, communication, and billing/claims you want to improve

After you answer questions like these, you can begin to address your specific EHR needs. Don't skimp on your list of EHR needs. If you do, you'll find that you might ignore some useful and necessary features of an EHR that could help you achieve everything from a higher quality of reporting to a more efficient workflow.

If you feel like your EHR needs list might get out of hand, try prioritizing your needs into Level 1, 2, and 3 categories. Level 1 are the "must-have" kind of needs, Level 2 are the necessary but less common needs or needs met less often, and Level 3 are the needs that you would like to meet, but can live without or find an alternate solution for.

Getting Everyone on Board

Face it — not everyone embraces technology. You'll find it isn't easy to coax tech-wary staff members from their paper-based shells. Change is difficult even for the most flexible individuals, and perhaps technological savvy isn't the issue, but the comfort of old workflows and processes is. Some people simply like the comfort of doing things the way they've always done them, which is perfectly normal. However, you have to increase their level of EHR comfort so they can approach the new adoption with confidence.

Have an open-door policy that allows employees to ask you anything about the move to EHR. Consider hosting frequent Q&A sessions or meeting with staff one-on-one to address their concerns. When in doubt, order in lunch and create a casual atmosphere to get everyone relaxed.

Start early in your project and involve your staff in the process. Give them some defined roles and encourage them to provide their feedback. As the implementation progresses, create opportunities for everyone to share their thoughts, concerns, and suggestions. You'll be surprised at some of the ideas that are presented and how much involving everyone improves your quality of care in ways you never imagined.

Keeping Track of All the Bells and Whistles

You review many potential EHR vendors as you narrow your search from hundreds of choices to just one final partner. Their sales reps tout all the features of their particular EHR (and trust us, there will be numerous features).

This is where knowing vendor capabilities can become very confusing. How do you remember what vendor offered the great code generator tool that you loved so much? Or which sales rep showed you the cool patient follow-up screens? Who knows — suddenly, all vendors and all EHR product capabilities look the same.

The key is to stay organized and have a system in place. Break out the spreadsheet or good old pen and paper so you can keep a running list of each potential EHR's features. Don't be afraid to take pictures of screens, materials, or even the vendors themselves; and make notes of key points or questions. That way, when you review your thoughts and sales information, you have a physical reminder of what you liked about each individual vendor offering. Don't forget that many tools are available from your Regional Extension Center (REC) and industry associations.

Your Regional Extension Center has done some due diligence in narrowing the field of choices and may provide a shortlist of vendors that can meet your needs. American EHR Partners (`www.americanehr.com`), founded by the American College of Physicians (ACP) in partnership with many other professional organizations, offers an EHR vendor directory, comparison engine, user ratings, and an automated request for information (RFI).

Getting and Keeping the Patient Involved

Patient engagement is key to your overall success, and a few obstacles likely lie in that path to success. Initially, many of your patients may have shared concerns about the security and privacy of their new electronic records. No one wants their patients to mistrust them, and that's why assuring your patients of reliable security is paramount to the success of your EHR implementation. Be proactive and offer information about the safety and security of patient records in various ways so you reach everyone who visits your office. Answer patient questions and concerns about security in person, via e-mail, via paper mailing, or any other way that makes your patient feel more comfortable about the state of EHR security.

Keep your patient information initiatives simple, direct, and focused on how the EHR will (or won't) change the patient experience. Create easy-to-read brochures that are free of technical jargon, keep in-person demonstrations short and targeted to specific patient concerns or questions, and offer tools that are easy for patients to access, like an online FAQ.

Dealing with Hardware Support and Reliability

You probably thought that because you have a big contract with an EHR vendor and that vendor is supporting your software that your computers and devices are covered, too. Unfortunately, more often than not, that's not the case. And now so many of your key clinical functions including simply accessing the patient record, filling prescriptions, and documenting your patient communications are tied inexorably to your hardware and network connectivity. Any small problem can have a major impact on your workflow efficiency or, even worse, patient safety.

Generally, most practices don't have the in-house resources to deal with the maintenance and troubleshooting for hardware devices. Here's how to deal with troubleshooting:

- ✔ Review any existing contracts you may have with a local store. See whether you need to expand these contracts to cover any new devices and services.

- ✔ Negotiate the services at the time of purchase to get the best deal. Many of the hardware suppliers, such as Dell, Hewlett-Packard, and Fujitsu, offer support services for a fee.

- ✔ See whether your EHR vendor can provide the hardware support and bundle the costs in your overall maintenance bill.

Receiving the Right Amount and Type of Training

Successful training is the key to your EHR success. But you can't exactly close the office for a week or two while employees acclimate to the new system. This is, after all, a business, so you have to find a way to complete training while still attending to the day-to-day needs of patients. Also, different users need different types of training. Some of your staff or colleagues may have very little experience with computers and will require some basic computer skills training in addition to the substantial EHR training.

If your EHR vendor or consultant feels confident that he can train your staff in a couple days, closing for a short time might be in your best interests. If so, notify your clients ahead of time and find a way to rotate staff during those two or three days so you still have someone to answer the phone, return calls, and manage care for any patients currently in the hospital. Another option is, of course, to train staff while the office remains open and (for the most part) fully functional, or conduct training before or after clinic hours. This, too, requires planning so the patients don't feel the weight of missing staff during their visits. Most organizations reduce the number of patients they see during the training period to account for any initial workflow inefficiencies. Ask your vendor rep for insight into his experience with how offices addressed training issues.

Knowing What Questions to Ask Vendors

You haven't done this before; how are you supposed to know what to ask the vendors? Well, now is the time to exercise that critical-thinking muscle. You can't always count on EHR vendors to provide you with all the answers upfront. Keep a running list of vendor questions handy while you research each product of interest and narrow your search results.

At minimum, you need to ask the vendor rep questions about how EHR addresses your specific needs, situations, or concerns about the following areas:

✔ **Front office functions**

- Intake

- Scheduling functionality

- Follow-up features

- Multi-stakeholder interactions, such as labs, pharmacies, and specialists

- Billing and coding accessibility

✔ **Nursing and medical assistant needs**

- Information capture

- Vitals functionality

- Ease and method of entering information, such as touchscreen, drop boxes, and so on

- Accessing and comparing patient history

✔ **Physician requirements**

- Method of transcription

- Accessibility of past interactions, lab results, and medications

- Functionality concerning information sharing

✒ **Patient concerns**

- Security and privacy

- Prescription accessibility

- Long-term management of their own care

✒ **ARRA and Meaningful Use reporting and readiness**

- Certification status and ability to meet 2011, 2013, and 2015 requirements

- Recourse if the product doesn't meet these requirements now or in the future

After you have some of those questions in mind, think about specific concerns that your staff or patients may be raising, and then add those to the mix. See Chapter 6 for a whole host of key questions and topics to review with your vendor partners.

Getting the Support You Need

Support doesn't end the week after you go-live. Support involves fixing issues that arise after the go-live and training on new functionality or features that you never actually figured out how to use. You can make sure your staff and you are on the cutting edge of the latest medical IT developments by taking part in continuing EHR education. Because you've chosen an EHR vendor who offers updated training over time (you did, right?), she will likely keep you informed of any new training she offers. Many vendors also keep you informed of training offerings from outside companies or organizations that might be applicable to your particular situation.

The system will break, or at least parts of it will; we know you were hoping that would never occur. Sometimes this happens after an upgrade from the vendor disrupts a system feature that was working. Other times, the system doesn't process information correctly based on design decisions or a change in your workflow or interfaces. Therefore, you need a plan to address and resolve all system issues. While you go through the selection and contracting process, work with the vendor to establish clear rules on how he'll support you. How fast will he respond to your calls or e-mails? How will he guarantee resolution to your problems? What additional resources is he willing to contribute to help you the most? Collaboratively decide on a process and expectations — and get it in writing as part of your Service Level Agreement (SLA) and contract.

Quelling a Revolt

You may never have a repeat of *Mutiny on the Bounty,* but every implementation has at least one mini-revolt. You have to respond to the issues and get everyone focused on doing the right thing. Sometimes these uprisings occur early in the process before you've really even started. Someone may push a little to see whether this EHR thing is really going to happen. Be ready to respond with a clear rationale for proceeding and a detailed plan to be successful.

A common time for stress and a potential revolt is at the go-live. Everyone's been trained, the vendor rep has officially left the building, and your paper files are somewhere in a storage facility in Schenectady. You're going live, baby! You have waited months (maybe years) for this moment, and there's no going back to the world of file folders and sticky notes. Now, the key is to make sure no one freaks out.

Many people experience a bit of EHR panic. They may forget something they learned in training and then proceed to forget everything else, or they may freeze the first time they have to do the dog and pony show of demonstrating an EHR function in front of a patient. Hey, we're all human, and it's normal and natural to feel a bit nervous about something new.

Keep your cool, and the rest of the staff is likely to do the same. You can maintain calm during go-live by giving people the tools they need to get over their initial EHR concerns. Keep training manuals handy, create short lists of the top ten EHR tasks, provide everyone with vendor rep and trainer contact information, and make yourself (or any other EHR point person) available to answer questions throughout the go-live period.

 Clear your schedule or reduce your personal workload during go-live week so you can assist fellow staffers with questions or concerns. You can also make sure that everyone feels connected as you move through the go-live process by offering open forums to discuss EHR issues and strategies. Allow time at regular staff meetings to answer EHR questions or even take everyone out to lunch for a casual debriefing session. The clinical champion (you) may want to continue with a reduced patient load for a few weeks until your practice is comfortable with using an EHR.

Designing a Long-Term EHR Strategy

You may be tempted to focus solely on the complexities of the go-live and not think much beyond that moment. However, the world keeps turning, healthcare regulations keep changing, and your EHR needs to evolve with those changes.

You'll hire new people, perhaps add a physician, change relationships with outside specialists or hospitals, and lose some people to retirement or job change. So, when you envision how EHR will take you into the coming years, consider how you'll address the ever-changing face of your staff.

Patients change as well, as do their needs. Like most medical professionals, you probably subscribe to numerous publications, e-mail lists, and professional organizations. Keep abreast of changing patient needs in terms of condition and disease management; communication issues; and, as always, emerging privacy issues so you can make sure you update how EHR interacts with this vital group of stakeholders. Remember that the go-live is just the beginning, and your successful EHR journey is a long and winding road. Keep your head up and continually work on improving the care you provide your patients by leveraging this new tool at your disposal.

Work with your vendor at the onset of implementation to create a framework for your long-term EHR strategy. You can make plans to review your needs on a regular basis (once or twice a year) and consult with your vendor to find solutions that keep you current in the world of healthcare IT. Make plans for continuing education for your employees, and find out how you can best stay abreast of new legislation and policy that might affect how you use the EHR. Remember that this is a long-term commitment, so go ahead and make a 5- or 10-year plan. You'll be glad you did.

Chapter 19

Ten Questions to Ask (And Answer)

In This Chapter
▶ Determining practice needs
▶ Creating a must-have list of features and services
▶ Engaging patients in their care

*Y*ou probably have a lot of questions about your impending EHR adoption and implementation. That's perfectly natural and, truth be told, keep questioning and finding out more information. We encourage you to ask (and in many cases, answer) these top ten questions. You'll certainly come up with more must-answer tidbits on your own, but here are some of the biggies you need to have at the top of your list.

Why Are You Doing This, and What Does This Practice Need?

Before you rush into your own implementation, you have to know why you're embarking on such a laborious effort. Although other practices and organizations have a variety of reasons, you need to understand which ones matter to you. What questions are you trying to answer, and what problems are you trying to remedy? Are you trying to improve patient outcomes, save money, comply with federal mandates, and receive stimulus funding or some other reason? You can look at other offices and try to duplicate their efforts and adopt their rationale for implementing EHR. In the end, you have to determine what your specific reasons and drivers are for starting this journey.

How Much Will EHR Adoption and Implementation Cost?

You need two things for EHR adoption and implementation: money and people. Yes, you have to spend real, physical money to purchase EHR software and have a real-live vendor rep at hand. You didn't think that EHR just grows on trees, did you? You need to have a clear picture of your EHR budget before you get too involved in shopping for a vendor. You also need to know what you hope to get in return for your investment (see Chapter 5). Work with your potential vendor reps to get a firm feel for both the initial and ongoing costs of

- ✔ Hardware
- ✔ Software
- ✔ Interfaces
- ✔ Other systems
- ✔ Loss in revenue because of lower productivity
- ✔ Training and support
- ✔ Software maintenance
- ✔ Upgrades

Try to factor in how incentive payments or penalties might affect your overall bottom line to get a truer picture of your EHR adoption and implementation financial plan.

How Do You Qualify for Incentives?

At the end of this, the government wants to write you a nice big check — that's not something you hear every day — but it may be something you hear more often after you get that new EHR up and running. Getting everyone on board with EHR is a government priority, so if you're using EHR under the specs of Meaningful Use, there's incentive money to be had. If you're an eligible professional who qualifies for Medicare or Medicaid payments through Meaningful Use of a certified EHR system, you can score up to five years' worth of incentive payments.

To receive the incentive payments, you need to meet the Meaningful Use criteria determined by the Centers for Medicare & Medicaid Services (CMS) and then demonstrate your compliance. Initially, CMS may just require an *attestation* (indicates that you meet the criteria) from you, but you may be subject to an audit or review to assure that you've met each criterion. Fortunately, resources can help you both meet the criteria and apply for your payment. Make sure to review Chapter 3 and look into how Regional Extension Centers, quality organizations, and your local hospitals can provide assistance.

If you're employed by a hospital system, clinic/group practice, corporate entity, or larger organization, your employment agreement or contract likely stipulates that the federal incentive dollars will be paid to the organization you work for, or contract to, and not to individual physicians. The big questions is, "Did your organization pay for your EHR or did you?" If your organization covered most of the costs, it's likely that the incentive payments will be used to defray those costs or cover costs of upgrades or additional training that you may need to meet Meaningful Use guidelines.

What Are Your Must-Have EHR Services and Features?

This question really goes hand-in-hand with your overall list of needs. After you determine what you and your staff need to get out of the EHR experience, you can create a firm list of your must-have needs. Consider these your *deal breakers* — if they aren't available, move on to another potential vendor.

To qualify for the Medicare or Medicaid incentives, your EHR must be certified by the Office of the National Coordinator-Authorized Testing and Certification Body (ONC-ATCB). A Certified Health Products List (CHPL) will contain all EHR vendor systems that are certified to meet Meaningful Use. For more information on certification and testing bodies, go to http://healthit.hhs.gov/certification or http://healthit.hhs.gov/ATCBs.

You may find it useful to create a multitiered listing of the services and features you most want the new EHR to have from the top down. You can create categories based on these priorities:

- **Non-negotiable:** These are absolute must-haves. Either you get them or you walk. For example, one of these must be that the system is certified to meet Meaningful Use to qualify for federal incentives.

- **Need it:** These are primary must-have services or features that you require on a daily basis. They are at the top of your must-have list, but you're willing to find alternatives to satisfy these needs as long as they are met somehow.

- **Want it:** These are services or features that would enhance your overall EHR experience, but you can possibly live without them. However, you will fast-track any vendor who offers them to the top of your contender list.

- **Window shopping:** These are services or features that would be wonderful to have, but you can live without them. But wouldn't they be nice?

Some vendors offer a guarantee, so push them a little and see whether they'll put their own money where their mouth is and help you get beyond installing the system to achieving Meaningful Use.

How Will Your Workflows Change?

In theory, you're getting EHR to reduce your daily interaction with and dependence on paper records. In practice, you're completely changing the way you do business each day. From the smallest details (how the front office staff scans insurance cards) to global issues (how prescriptions are managed), you can alter your workflows in a way that improved the office experience for both patients and employees.

We discuss what to do post-implementation in Chapter 8. Before you do any implementing, though, have an idea of how your pre-EHR practice already works. Then find ways you can improve on those longstanding processes post-EHR. Think about what functions will change and whether they need improvement. After you know these things, you can work with your employees and a new, enthusiastic vendor rep to design EHR that best answers your organization's workflow needs.

What Is the Best Way to Involve and Educate Your Patients?

Your patients are the true end consumers of EHR. After all, the management of their health records makes EHR what it is. As such, you have to keep them in the loop about the new electronic form in which their health records now exist. You have two major hurdles to overcome here: security concerns and fear of technology. To alleviate both, consider offering patient education in multiple formats so that you reach each patient in the way that he or she is most comfortable. For example, as we mention in Chapter 9, don't just include a flyer about the changes with a patient's latest bill. Instead, train office staff to explain what they're doing with patients during their day-to-day interactions. Consider offering patient education in other formats, such as

✔ E-mail updates, blasts, or newsletters

✔ Twitter feeds

✔ Instant messages

✔ Print media (brochures, flyers, or booklets)

✔ Video podcasts

✔ DVDs or CDs

✔ Personal tutorials

✔ Social networking pages

✔ Corporate Web site FAQs

✔ Meet and greet training sessions with staff or physicians

Regardless of how you communicate EHR information to your patients, keep the focus on what EHR can do for them. Make EHR fun and show them how to manage their healthcare using your shiny, new EHR tools.

How Do You Plan a Smooth Go-Live?

Planning and organization are your keys to go-live success. Following a detailed plan and staying organized are the keystones to a successful go-live. You'll still have a hiccup here and there, but you'll be prepared and have a plan for whatever comes up.

As part of your all-important plan, several focus areas are of key importance:

✔ **Support:** Have a schedule for who provides support and where he or she is; factor in who might now need the most assistance.

✔ **Communication:** Keep everyone apprised of what's going on, including your staff, colleagues, and patients.

✔ **Leadership:** Everyone needs to know who the go-to person (probably you) is, and keep your cool during the event. People gravitate toward strong leaders and stay calm if the chain of command is steady and decisive.

✔ **Patient schedule:** Keep the schedule light if possible, and if you can, limit any new patients or major procedures during the first week or so.

✔ **Little things:** Don't forget the important things, such as food and coffee and saying thank you. You'll be surprised at how a few words of encouragement can go such a long way in helping people cope with the stress of a go-live.

What Kind of Ongoing Support Can You Expect from the Vendor?

Think of ongoing support in two categories: technical and education/innovation. Your vendor needs to cover you in both areas and help you keep things running in terms of hardware/software and keeping your staff on the cutting edge of EHR functionality.

In addition to the general upkeep of the hardware, make sure to have a firm understanding of the issue resolution process because, at times, the system will either break or not work the way that you expect it to. Your vendor is a key resource in helping to fix any software issues. Work with him to agree upon a process to report issues, monitor progress, and ultimately, resolve the problems.

During contract negotiations, make sure you carefully read (and modify as needed) the vendor Service Level Agreement (SLA). The SLA should clearly define the level of service you are to receive, describe the terms (say response time), and specify any additional costs. Your contract or SLA should also stipulate any repercussions or recourse you have if your contracted service levels aren't met.

When you're ready to turn on EHR and go-live, the vendor will likely have resources to support you and your staff. Vendor support strategies vary in terms of how long the vendor remains onsite, when he or she comes back, what type of resources he or she uses, and what ongoing support he or she will provide. Some vendors are not providing any onsite support for very small practices. The vendors want you to be self-sufficient. No matter how well a vendor performs on day one, the vendor won't always be perfect.

How Can EHR Help Patients with Their Care?

Gone are the days of patients hauling around file folders full of charts, lab results, immunization records, and prescription lists (sound familiar?). Currently, a patient uses two main tools to help manage and contribute to their care: the patient portal and the personal health record (PHR). Some patients may use the PHR available to them via their employer, payer, and so on. Our focus in this book is on the patient portal because it's generally developed and maintained by your EHR vendor.

Patients can make use of a patient portal to provide key information to their physicians and potentially communicate using secure messaging. In this way, patients can be active participants in the management of their healthcare right along with physicians, nurses, practitioners, pharmacists, specialists, and even lab techs. Portals may also allow patients to

✔ Complete forms online prior to an office or hospital visit

✔ Request prescription refills

✔ View their medical records

✔ Review billing statements

✔ Set up online payments

✔ View lab results or diagnostic images

✔ Schedule or change appointments

✔ Set up conversations with providers

✔ Update certain clinical information

✔ E-mail or instant message providers

Patients who can't make regular visits to your office can also take part in remote patient monitoring (RPM). This is a great tool for those who have chronic conditions in need of constant monitoring. RPM allows health-care professionals to monitor patient vital signs, measure physiological responses, and communicate when physical distance prohibits office visits. RPM provides a cost benefit as well as improved quality to both practitioners and patients thanks to ease of reporting and quick delivery of information.

In addition to these cool tools (see Chapter 2), you can work with patients to enjoy the benefits of EHR, even if it's simply on an office visit level. You and your patients can look at charts, diagnostics, and images together, creating a more open environment for patient communication.

How Will EHR Benefit Your Practice?

This is the ultimate question to ask (and answer) yourself. Only one person — you — can truly offer the best answer here. Some benefits are obvious: less dependence on paper files, improved workflow, better quality of care, accuracy in billing and reimbursements, financial incentives . . . the list can go on. However, you, and only you, can mesh your needs/wants list with your must-have features and services list to see how EHR will truly benefit your unique clinical situation. Remember that realizing the benefits of your EHR implementation is a long journey. Your go-live isn't the end of the road — it's just the beginning. Here are some of the key steps:

✔ Identify areas of opportunity and expected benefit.

✔ Capture baseline measurements.

✔ Design the system, decision support, workflows, and content to support your benefits strategy.

✔ Use the system as designed (that means everyone, not just you).

✔ Measure your outcomes.

✔ Analyze the results.

✔ Refine the system and your processes to continually improve.

✔ Repeat the process.

Appendix A

Alphabet Soup

*T*he world of electronic health records has many acronyms floating around. For your reading and reference enjoyment, we present these acronyms in an easy-to-peruse alphabetized list. Enjoy your alphabet soup!

AAFP: American Association of Family Physicians. National medical society that serves as the primary professional, policy, and advocacy organization for family practice physicians.

AAP: American Academy of Pediatrics. National medical society that serves as the primary professional, policy, and advocacy organization for pediatricians.

ACMPE: The American College of Medical Practice Executives. An arm of the Medical Group Management Association (MGMAS) that sets standards for the industry and promotes the professional development of PM leaders. *See also* MGMA.

ACO: Accountable Care Organization. A new model emerging as a result of health reform where an organization that includes primary care physicians, specialists, and at least one hospital, share responsibility for the quality and the cost of care received by patients of the organization.

ACP: American College of Physicians. National medical society that serves as the primary professional, policy, and advocacy organization for internists. ACP established AmericanEHR Partners, a program focused on assisting physicians to adopt Health Information Technology.

AHQA: American Health Quality Association. An umbrella organization representing a national network of community-based Quality Improvement Organizations (QIOs) and other professionals working to improve the quality of healthcare.

AHRQ: Agency for Healthcare Research and Quality National Resource Center for Health Information Technology

AMA: American Medical Association. National professional, policy, and advocacy organization for physicians, residents, fellows, and medical students.

ANSI: American National Standards Institute

AQA: Ambulatory Care Quality Alliance. A wide-reaching group that includes several stakeholder groups who agree on ways to measure performance and report their findings to consumers to improve patient outcomes.

ARRA: American Recovery and Reinvestment Act. Signed into law by President Obama in February 2009, ARRA was created in response to the economic crisis to help spur recovery by increasing economic activity and investments, create new jobs, save existing jobs, and create more account-ability in government spending. The act increases federal funds for various programs (like healthcare) by $224 billion and frees $275 billion for federal contracts, grants, and loans, some of which affect the healthcare sector.

ASP: Application service provider. The ASP model is used when an external party maintains and stores your practice's data.

ATA: American Telemedicine Association

BPR: Business Process Reengineering. The analysis and redesign of work-flows between enterprises.

CAST: Center for Aging Services Technologies

CCHIT: Certification Commission for Health Information Technology. A not-for-profit group whose mission is to accelerate the adoption of health IT by improving quality, safety, efficiency, and access. CCHIT was (founded in 2004) primarily providing certifications for EHRs since 2006. Eligible profes-sionals who use products certified by CCHIT's ONC-ATCB 2011/2012 certi-fication program and meet Meaningful Use criteria can qualify for federal incentives from Medicare or Medicaid.

CHPL: ONC's Certified Health IT Product List

CMS: Centers for Medicare and Medicaid Studies

CPeH: The Consumer Partnership for eHealth. A non-partisan coalition led by the National Partnership for Women and Families, has been working since 2005 to ensure that health IT adoption efforts meet the needs of patients and their families. Several organizations, including big players (AARP, AFL-CIO, Center for Medical Consumers, and the National Consumers League) are part of this coalition that works at national and local levels with a membership that represents more than 127 million Americans.

CPT: Current procedural technology. A listing of standardized alphanumeric codes that medical coders use to report services.

DIM: Document management system. Indexes, stores, and manages any scanned or faxed items included in your EHR.

EHR: Electronic Health Record. An electronic record of health-related information on an individual that conforms to nationally recognized interoperability standards and that can be created, managed, and consulted by authorized clinicians and staff across more than one healthcare organization or department. *See also* EMR.

EMR: Electronic Medical Record. An electronic record of health-related information on an individual that can be created, gathered, managed, and consulted by authorized clinicians and staff within one healthcare organization. The term *EMR* has been used to refer to ambulatory electronic record systems, but *EHR* is becoming increasingly common in the ambulatory setting. *See also* EHR.

EPHI: Electronic Protected Health Information

eRx: Electronic prescribing (e-prescribing) allows you to send, confirm, and refill prescriptions safely and quickly to participating pharmacies online.

FACA: Federal Advisory Committee Act

HIE: Health information exchange. The exchange of health information across organizations, such as hospitals, ambulatory practices, testing organizations, or other local and regional systems.

HIPAA: Health Insurance Portability and Accountability Act. Among other duties, HIPAA mandates industry-wide standards for healthcare information on electronic billing and other processes.

HIMSS: Health Information Management and Systems Society. The biggest professional organization supporting the health IT community that includes membership from hospitals, health systems, and vendors.

HITECH: Health Information Technology for Economic and Clinical Health Act. The HITECH Act is largely concerned with privacy and security concerns that may arise from an electronic-based system.

HITSP: Healthcare Information Technology Standards Panel. Group that works in partnership with public and private healthcare sectors to create a set of standards that can enable operability among healthcare software applications.

HHS: The U.S. Department of Health and Human Services. The principal federal agency for protecting the health of Americans and providing essential human services. *See also* ONC.

HL7: Health Level Seven International. A not-for-profit organization that develops standards designed to create a framework for the use, exchange, sharing, and retrieval of electronic health information with the goal of supporting clinical practice management. *See also* IHE.

HMO: Health maintenance organization

HRSA: Heath Resources and Services Administration. The primary federal agency for improving access to healthcare services for people who are uninsured, isolated, or medically vulnerable.

ICD: International Classification of Diseases. A set of codes used by physicians, hospitals, and allied health workers to indicate diagnosis for all patient encounters. ICD9 (9th edition) and ICD9-CM (9th edition, clinical modifications) have been in use since 1979. The official compliance date for ICD10 (10th edition) has been pushed to October 1, 2013 and to January 1, 2012 for 5010 HIPAA transaction sets.

IHE: Integrating the Healthcare Enterprise. An initiative created by healthcare professionals to improve how computer systems in healthcare share information across applications, systems, stakeholders, and settings. IHE promotes the coordinated use of established standards, such as DICOM and HL7 to support standards-based, interoperable exchange of health information.

ICR: Intelligent Character Recognition. Reads written information, which could assist in collecting patient registration and history information.

IT: Information technology. Describes any technology used to create, store, view, exchange and utilize information and data. Might also be referred to as IS (information systems).

KLAS: Market research firm that publishes ratings of healthcare IT vendors.

MGMA: Medical Group Management Association. The premier membership association for professional administrators and leaders of medical group practices.

MIPPA: Medicare Improvements for Patients and Providers Act

NACHC: National Association of Community Health Centers

NCQA: National Committee for Quality Assurance. A private, 501(c)(3) not-for-profit organization dedicated to improving health care quality.

NGC: National Guideline Clearinghouse. A resource for the public so all stakeholder groups (patients in particular) can review evidence-based clinical practice guidelines.

NIST: The National Institute of Standards and Technology. An agency of the U.S. Department of Commerce that's involved in several levels of healthcare IT interoperability. The institute works with major standards development organizations, professional associations, and the public to promote safe standards-based solutions for the exchange of healthcare information.

NQF: National Quality Forum. A not-for-profit organization that seeks to create and implement a national strategy for quality measurement and reporting.

OCR: Optical Character Recognition. Reads machine-printed characters and letters, which could help determine paper document types and automatically match scanned documents with a patient's record and encounter

OMR: Optical Mark Recognition. Reads optical marks (such as checkmarks) on a form, which could assist in capturing patient histories.

ONC: Office of the National Coordinator for Health Information Technology. Under the umbrella of the Department of Health and Human Services (HHS), this group is charged with promoting the development of a nationwide health information technology infrastructure.

ONC-ATCB: ONC Accredited Testing and Certification Body. A practice must use an EHR certified by an ONC-ATCB to be eligible for incentives from Medicare or Medicaid.

QA: Quality assurance

QIO: Quality Improvement Organization. CMS contracts with one organization in each state/jurisdiction to serve as its QIO contractor. QIOs are private, mostly not-for-profit organizations, which are staffed by professionals to improve the effectiveness, efficiency, economy, and quality of services delivered to Medicare beneficiaries. Many QIOs are also serving as Regional Extension Centers (RECs).

P4P: Pay-for-performance. Programs created by healthcare payers to encourage physicians to follow evidence-based guidelines for preventive and chronic disease care measures.

PCPI: American Medical Association Physician Consortium for Performance Improvement. An AMA-sponsored group committed to improving quality of care and patient safety. This group develops, tests, and maintains evidence-based clinical performance standards.

PDCA: Plan-Do-Check-Act. A process improvement system that focuses on solving business process problems.

PHI: Protected health information. The Office of Civil Rights defines PHI as individually identifiable health information held or transmitted by a covered entity or its business associate, in any form or media, whether electronic, paper, or oral.

PHR: Personal health record. A record that keeps track of a patient's personal health history. Not to be confused with the EHR (which is the documentation of the healthcare provider), the PHR's content is owned and managed by the patient or patient's caregiver.

PM: Practice management. More than just managing how you use and share files, practice management involves people management, improving communication between staffers, creating stronger methods of communication with outside entities or patients, and setting up your office for financial success through accurate billing and coding.

POC: Point of care

REC: Regional Extension Center. Organization that's responsible for a specific geographic area and expected to support providers in achieving Meaningful Use.

RFI: Request for information

RHIO: Regional health information organization

ROI: Return on investment

RPM: Remote patient monitoring. Allows healthcare professionals to monitor patient vital signs, measure physiological responses, and communicate when physical distance prohibits office visits. Remote patient monitoring provides cost benefits and improved quality to practitioners and patients thanks to the ease of reporting and quick delivery of information.

SaaS: Software as a Service. A service delivery model where software deploys over the Internet to run on a local network or personal computer that's priced using a subscription or pay-as-you-go model. For EHRs, the term _SaaS_ and _ASP_ are often used interchangeably. **_See also_** ASP.

SLA: Service Level Agreement. Part of the contract terms and conditions from an EHR vendor that defines the level of service and costs that will be provided under the service contract.

TQM: Total Quality Management. Seeks to improve quality by ensuring compliance with internal requirements.

Appendix B

Regional Extension Centers

. . . .

*R*egional Extension Centers are being added on a daily basis. If you don't find one that services your area in the following list, check out www. HealthIT.hhs.gov/programs/REC/.

REC Name	State	Web Site
Alaska eHealth Network	AK	www.ak-ehealth.com
Alabama Regional Extension Center	AL	www.al-rec.org
HIT Arkansas	AR	www.hitarkansas.com
Arizona Health-e Connection (AzHeC)	AZ	www.azhec.org
CalHIPSO (North)	CA	www.calhipso.org
CalHIPSO (South)	CA	www.calhipso.org
CalOptima Foundation	CA	www.caloptima.org
HITEC-LA	CA	http://hitec-la.org
Colorado Regional Extension Center (CORHIO)	CO	www.corhio.org
eHealth Connecticut	CT	www.ehealthconnecticut. org
eHealth DC	DC	www.ehealthdc.org
National Indian Health Board (NIHB)	DC	www.nihb.org
Quality Insights of Delaware	DE	www.qide.org/de
Rural and North Florida Regional Extension Center	FL	www.chcalliance.org/ Services/egional ExtensionCenter.aspx
South Florida Regional Extension Center Collaborative	FL	www.southfloridarec.org
University of Central Florida	FL	www.med.ucf.edu/rec/

(continued)

REC Name	State	Web Site
University of South Florida	FL	http://health.usf.edu/paperfree/index.htm
Morehouse School of Medicine	GA	www.msm.edu/research/research_centersand institutes/research_cni_NCPC.aspx
Hawaii Health Information Exchange	HI	www.hhie.org
IFMC Health Information Technology Regional Extension Center (Iowa HITREC)	IA	www.IowaHITREC.org
Illinois Health Information Technology REC (Il-HITREC)	IL	www.ilhitrec.org
Chicago Health Information Technology REC (CHITREC)	IL	www.chitrec.org
Purdue University	IN	www.ihitec.purdue.edu
Kansas Foundation for Medical Care, Inc. (KFCM)	KS	www.kfmc.org/rec
University of Kentucky Research Foundation	KY	www2.ca.uky.edu
REC for Health IT in Mississippi	MS	www.eqhealthsolutions.com
Louisiana Health Care Quality Forum	LA	www.lhcqf.org
MA Technology Corporation	MA	http://masstech.org
Chesapeake Regional Information System for Our Patients	MD	www.crisphealth.org
HealthInfoNet	ME	www.hinfonet.org
Michigan Center for Effective IT Adoption (M-CEITA)	MI	www.mceita.org
Regional Extension Assistance Center for HIT (REACH)	MN	www.khareach.org
Missouri HIT Assistance Center	MO	www.assistancecenter.missouri.edu
Mountain Pacific Quality Health Foundation (MPQHF)	MT	www.mpqhf.org

REC Name	State	Web Site
University of North Carolina at Chapel Hill	NC	www.med.unc.edu/ahec
Wide River Technology Extension Center	NE	www.widerivertec.org
Massachusetts eHealth Collaborative	NH	www.maehc.org
New Jersey Institute of Technology	NJ	www.njit.edu
LCF Research	NM	www.lcfresearch.org
NYC REACH	NY	www.nycreach.org
New York eHealth Collaborative (NYeC)	NY	www.nyehealth.org
HealthBridge Inc.	OH, KY, IN	www.healthbridge.org
Ohio Health Information Partnership (OHIP)	OH	http://ohiponline.org
Oklahoma Foundation for Medical Quality (OFMQ)	OK	www.ofmq.com
O-HITEC	OR	http://o-hitec.org
Quality Insights of Pennsylvania East	PA	www.qipa.org/pa
Quality Insights of Pennsylvania West	PA	www.qipa.org/pa
Ponce School of Medicine	PR	www.psm.edu
Rhode Island Quality Institute	RI	www.riqi.org
South Carolina Research Foundation	SC	www.healthsciencessc.org
South Dakota REC (SD-REC)	SD	www.cahit.dsu.edu
Qsource	TN	www.tnrec.org
North Texas REC	TX	www.dfwhc.org
West Texas HIT REC (WT-HITREC)	TX	www.ttuhsc.edu
CentrEast REC	TX	http://centreastrec.org
University of Texas Health Science Center at Houston	TX	www.shis.uth.tmc.edu

(continued)

REC Name	State	Web Site
Health Insight	UT	www.healthinsight.org
VHQC (Virginia Health Quality Center)	VA	www.vhqc.org
Vermont IT Leaders	VT	www.vitl.net
WI-REC	WA	www.wirecqh.org
Wisconsin HIT Extension Center	WI	www.whitec.org
West Virginia Health Improvement	WV	www.wvhealthimprovement.org/wvhii/home.aspx

Appendix C

Medicare and Medicaid Incentives

*I*f you are an eligible professional who qualifies for Medicare or Medicaid payments through Meaningful Use of a certified EHR system, you can score up to five years' worth of incentive payments starting as early as 2011. Now, how much you can potentially receive depends on the year you begin qualifying. Here is the payment breakdown:

- ✔ If your first qualifying year is 2011 or 2012, you can receive up to $18,000 in EHR-related incentives.

- ✔ If you don't apply until 2013, the annual incentive payment limits in the first through fourth years are $15,000, $12,000, $8000, and $4000, respectively, for a total of $39,000.

- ✔ The maximum amount of incentive payments you can receive under Medicare is $44,000. That's not chump change.

- ✔ If you meet the Medicaid patient volume requirements, you can receive a higher potential first year payment, which is an incentive payment of $21,250 and a total of $63,750. Your timing to receive this payment is limited by your state's level of readiness to process Medicaid payments for Meaningful Use, so it will be important to check with your specific state's Medicaid office or REC to obtain this information.

The following tables show how the incentives and potential reductions are expected to work from 2011–2017.

Medicare Incentive Payment Schedule

First Payment Year	First Payment Year Amount, and Subsequent Payment Amounts in Following Years	Reduction in Fee Schedule for Non-Adoption/Use
2011	$18k, $12k, $8k, $4k, and $2k	$0
2012	$18k, $12k, $8k, $4k, and $2k	$0
2013	$15k, $12k, $8k, and $4k	$0
2014	$12k ,$8k, and $4k	$0
2015	$0	−1% of Medicare fee schedule
2016	$0	−2% of Medicare fee schedule
2017 and thereafter	$0	−3% of Medicare fee schedule

Medicaid Incentive Payment Schedule

First Payment Year	First Payment Year Amount, and Subsequent Payment Amounts in Following Years*	Reduction in Fee Schedule for Non-Adoption/Use
2011	$21,250, $8.5k, $8.5k, $8.5k, and $8.5k	$0
2012	$21,250, $8.5k, $8.5k, $8.5k, and $8.5k	$0
2013	$21,250, $8.5k, $8.5k, $8.5k, and $8.5k	$0
2014	$21,250, $8.5k, $8.5k, $8.5k, and $8.5k	$0
2015	$21,250, $8.5k, $8.5k, $8.5k, and $8.5k	$0
2016	$21,250, $8.5k, $8.5k, $8.5k, and $8.5k	$0
2017 and thereafter	$0	$0

Index

• U •

• V •

Apple & Macs

iPad For Dummies
978-0-470-58027-1

iPhone For Dummies,
4th Edition
978-0-470-87870-5

MacBook For Dummies, 3rd
Edition
978-0-470-76918-8

Mac OS X Snow Leopard For
Dummies
978-0-470-43543-4

Business

Bookkeeping For Dummies
978-0-7645-9848-7

Job Interviews
For Dummies,
3rd Edition
978-0-470-17748-8

Resumes For Dummies,
5th Edition
978-0-470-08037-5

Starting an
Online Business
For Dummies,
6th Edition
978-0-470-60210-2

Stock Investing
For Dummies,
3rd Edition
978-0-470-40114-9

Successful
Time Management
For Dummies
978-0-470-29034-7

Computer Hardware

BlackBerry
For Dummies,
4th Edition
978-0-470-60700-8

Computers For Seniors
For Dummies,
2nd Edition
978-0-470-53483-0

PCs For Dummies,
Windows
7 Edition
978-0-470-46542-4

Laptops For Dummies,
4th Edition
978-0-470-57829-2

Cooking & Entertaining

Cooking Basics
For Dummies,
3rd Edition
978-0-7645-7206-7

Wine For Dummies,
4th Edition
978-0-470-04579-4

Diet & Nutrition

Dieting For Dummies,
2nd Edition
978-0-7645-4149-0

Nutrition For Dummies,
4th Edition
978-0-471-79868-2

Weight Training
For Dummies,
3rd Edition
978-0-471-76845-6

Digital Photography

Digital SLR Cameras &
Photography For Dummies,
3rd Edition
978-0-470-46606-3

Photoshop Elements 8
For Dummies
978-0-470-52967-6

Gardening

Gardening Basics
For Dummies
978-0-470-03749-2

Organic Gardening
For Dummies,
2nd Edition
978-0-470-43067-5

Green/Sustainable

Raising Chickens
For Dummies
978-0-470-46544-8

Green Cleaning
For Dummies
978-0-470-39106-8

Health

Diabetes For Dummies,
3rd Edition
978-0-470-27086-8

Food Allergies
For Dummies
978-0-470-09584-3

Living Gluten-Free
For Dummies,
2nd Edition
978-0-470-58589-4

Hobbies/General

Chess For Dummies,
2nd Edition
978-0-7645-8404-6

Drawing
Cartoons & Comics
For Dummies
978-0-470-42683-8

Knitting For Dummies,
2nd Edition
978-0-470-28747-7

Organizing
For Dummies
978-0-7645-5300-4

Su Doku For Dummies
978-0-470-01892-7

Home Improvement

Home Maintenance
For Dummies,
2nd Edition
978-0-470-43063-7

Home Theater
For Dummies,
3rd Edition
978-0-470-41189-6

Living the
Country Lifestyle
All-in-One
For Dummies
978-0-470-43061-3

Solar Power Your Home
For Dummies,
2nd Edition
978-0-470-59678-4

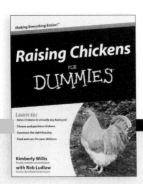

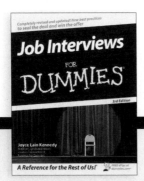

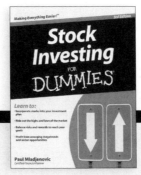

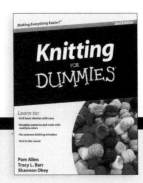

Internet

Blogging For Dummies,
3rd Edition
978-0-470-61996-4

eBay For Dummies,
6th Edition
978-0-470-49741-8

Facebook For Dummies,
3rd Edition
978-0-470-87804-0

Web Marketing
For Dummies,
2nd Edition
978-0-470-37181-7

WordPress
For Dummies,
3rd Edition
978-0-470-59274-8

Language & Foreign Language

French For Dummies
978-0-7645-5193-2

Italian Phrases
For Dummies
978-0-7645-7203-6

Spanish For Dummies,
2nd Edition
978-0-470-87855-2

Spanish
For Dummies,
Audio Set
978-0-470-09585-0

Math & Science

Algebra I
For Dummies,
2nd Edition
978-0-470-55964-2

Biology For Dummies,
2nd Edition
978-0-470-59875-7

Calculus For Dummies
978-0-7645-2498-1

Chemistry For Dummies
978-0-7645-5430-8

Microsoft Office

Excel 2010 For Dummies
978-0-470-48953-6

Office 2010 All-in-One
For Dummies
978-0-470-49748-7

Office 2010 For Dummies,
Book + DVD Bundle
978-0-470-62698-6

Word 2010 For Dummies
978-0-470-48772-3

Music

Guitar For Dummies,
2nd Edition
978-0-7645-9904-0

iPod & iTunes For
Dummies, 8th Edition
978-0-470-87871-2

Piano Exercises
For Dummies
978-0-470-38765-8

Parenting & Education

Parenting For Dummies,
2nd Edition
978-0-7645-5418-6

Type 1 Diabetes
For Dummies
978-0-470-17811-9

Pets

Cats For Dummies,
2nd Edition
978-0-7645-5275-5

Dog Training For Dummies,
3rd Edition
978-0-470-60029-0

Puppies For Dummies,
2nd Edition
978-0-470-03717-1

Religion & Inspiration

The Bible For Dummies
978-0-7645-5296-0

Catholicism For Dummies
978-0-7645-5391-2

Women in the Bible
For Dummies
978-0-7645-8475-6

Self-Help & Relationship

Anger Management
For Dummies
978-0-470-03715-7

Overcoming Anxiety
For Dummies,
2nd Edition
978-0-470-57441-6

Sports

Baseball
For Dummies,
3rd Edition
978-0-7645-7537-2

Basketball
For Dummies,
2nd Edition
978-0-7645-5248-9

Golf For Dummies,
3rd Edition
978-0-471-76871-5

Web Development

Web Design
All-in-One
For Dummies
978-0-470-41796-6

Web Sites
Do-It-Yourself
For Dummies,
2nd Edition
978-0-470-56520-9

Windows 7

Windows 7
For Dummies
978-0-470-49743-2

Windows 7
For Dummies,
Book + DVD Bundle
978-0-470-52398-8

Windows 7 All-in-One
For Dummies
978-0-470-48763-1

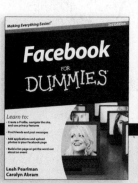
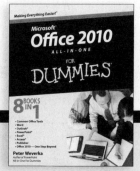
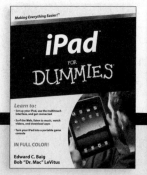
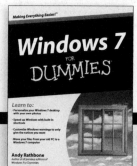

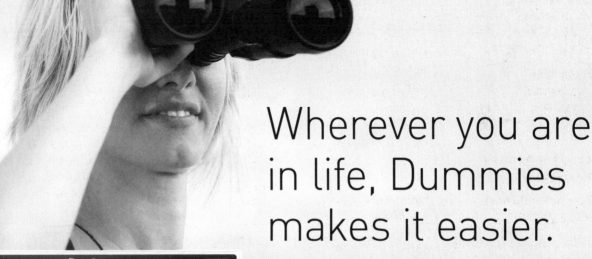
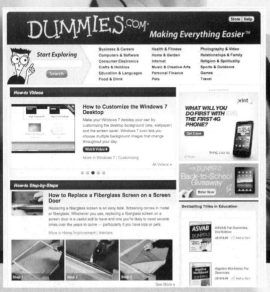
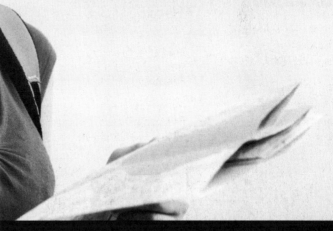

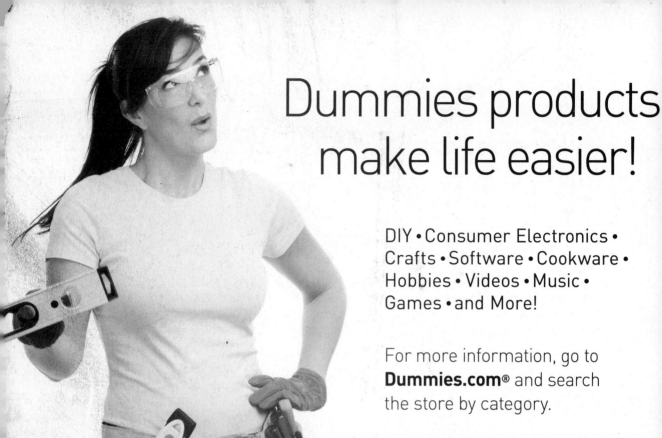
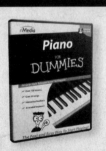
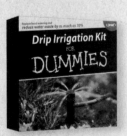
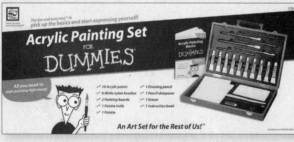
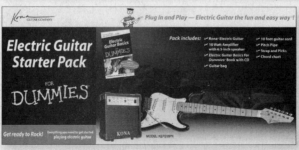
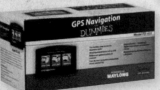
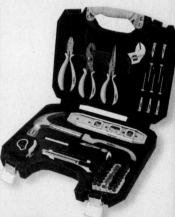
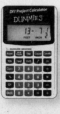
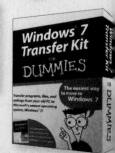
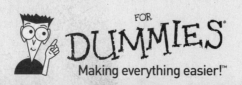